ORTH. 47

D1643649

THE
BACK
BOOK

Healing
the Hurt
in Your
Lower Back

THE BACK BOOK

Healing the Hurt in Your Lower Back

MAGGIE LETTVIN

Drawings
by Ruth McCambridge

Foreword
by Ralph H. Bender, M.D.

SOUVENIR PRESS

First published in the U.S.A. by
Houghton Mifflin Company

First British Edition published 1978 by
Souvenir Press Ltd, 43 Great Russell Street London WC1B 3PA

ISBN 0 285 62323 0

Printed and bound in Great Britain by
REDWOOD BURN LIMITED
Trowbridge & Esher

I have said to Charlotte Michaelson
in many a different way
day after day
"I could never have done this without you"
and it has always been true.

Acknowledgments

I AM LUCKY to have a community of my teachers and student teachers at the Massachusetts Institute of Technology and am grateful for their continuing criticism and help in the development of this material on low back pain. They are:

Leslie Brown
Suzanne Brown
Sheila Filippone
Richard Gardner
Leonard Goodman
Eleonor E. Hellman-Sogin

Betty Brack Maltas
Nancy R. Margolin
Ronald E. Parker
Mindy Rauch
Helli Sharfman
Shirley Noakes Zumino

Foreword

WHY ANOTHER BOOK on backache? The bookstalls are already flooded with volumes promising to explain, control, and cure ever-present miseries. The methods proposed deal with cures relying on programs as varied as mind control, diet, or extensive exercise regimes. What has been left out?

Back pain is a major source of difficulty for increasing numbers of people in our society. There are multiple causes. However, there are common features that make it desirable to form a unified approach to rehabilitation once specific problems have been defined and controlled.

One area in which many physicians fail when treating patients with back problems is in explaining adequately the objectives and the mechanics of the rehabilitative process. We tend to be concerned with diagnosis and with the control of acute pain, but we rarely have the time or patience to instruct our patients in their role in achieving maximum recovery.

Rehabilitation requires mobilization and gradual strengthening of the tissues that support and move the spine. These include the soft tissues of the back and also the muscles of the abdomen and buttocks. Maggie has demonstrated that rehabilitation can be achieved in a simple, logical manner. It is not necessary to employ extensive gadgetry, or endless exercise variations. It is necessary to learn an effective program and to follow it. Maggie has designed such a program and has been able to describe it in a manner that can be easily understood and followed. The written descriptions anticipate questions that might arise, and emphasize the sensations that can alert one to whether the exercise is being performed accurately, sufficiently, or excessively. The diagrams simply and accurately reflect and supplement the text. Both the diagrams and text emphasize the importance of attention to detail and to the sensations of discomfort.

Why another book on backache? We need one that can be used by nearly anyone with back pain to learn to return to an effective functional status. We need one that works!

Ralph H. Bender, M.D.

Contents

Introduction

IT IS EASY to say that back troubles happen because we stand upright. But other beings also get back trouble; for example, horses get swayback, and dachshunds have problems very like ours. While many people complain of low back pain, the important thing is that just as many and more go to old age with only an occasional twinge or a short episode. Because it is possible to live an active, upright life without continual back problems, we should not look at the disease as a necessary burden that can't be helped. Instead, we should find what differences there are among the ways of using the back. Often when we see what causes pain, we can change conditions enough to relieve it.

If we look on our bodies as machines, we can most often spot the sources of back trouble quickly and without complex arguments. We differ from ordinary machines, however, in one marvelous respect — we are self-repairing. Many troubles can be reversed simply by changing how we handle ourselves. The parts grow to adjust, and in a while we have a rebuilt body.

The way we live almost insures that if we injure our backs we will have a hard time getting better. Our sitting habits, our fashions in clothing and furniture, the hard pavements of the city, and the mental tensions that are reflected in general muscle tensions, all tend to make a sore back worse.

Recovery from most back injuries places the burden more upon the patient than on the doctor. At best, the doctor can only guide us to our recovery. But he cannot do so if how we act between visits goes against the thrust of his advice and treatment. Often such improper action comes from our not knowing enough about our own backs to tell what will worsen them.

The crude mechanics of the back are not hard to understand. Most of the time we can see easily what influences hurt us and what changes lessen that hurt. Then we can help to plan our own relief and to design our own healing. That is what this book is about.

xiii

THE BACK BOOK

Healing the Hurt in Your Lower Back

ONE

Understanding Your Own Pain

When you are in pain it is hard to be specific about the pain — to know what it comes from, what brings it on, exactly where it is, what makes it continue.

It is important to keep an account of your back pain so as to compare one time with another. Only you can tell if you are getting better or worse. But you must have a reliable way of telling. Everyone has changing moods and a selective memory. For example, a depressed person remembers mostly suffering and an elated person remembers cheerful events.

Therefore you can't really trust your memory. You need a chart of what hurts, when, how much, and what caused the hurt. From the chart you can then tell if you are getting better or not, what habits you may have to change, what positions you must avoid, what postures are most comfortable. How quickly you heal depends greatly on how little damage you do to yourself while healing. And every time you start up a severe pain you delay your recovery. If you know what to avoid, and train yourself to avoid it, your back heals and you recover much sooner.

The questionnaire and the Pain–Time Charts in this chapter will uncover a lot of information you were never aware of. Filling in the charts and questionnaire will help you detect facts about your pain so that you can decide upon the best possible remedies for your own back.

1

Questionnaire

1. Are you under a doctor's care now for this problem? __
2. Are you in constant pain? __
3. When did the pain start? _____
4. How long have you had it? _____
5. Was the pain caused by: Is the pain:
   - a. poor posture? __   a. seasonal? __
   - b. overweight? __   b. weather-related? __
   - c. pregnancy? __   c. stress-related? __
   - d. menopause? __   d. other? Be specific. __
   - e. accident? __   _____
   - f. illness? __   _____
   - g. disease? __
6. Does another member of your family have a low back problem? __
   Who? _____
7. Is the pain sharp? __ dull? __ intermittent? __
8. Where on your back do you feel pain? (Draw on sketch.)
9. Is it a radiating pain? __
10. Where does the pain radiate, or move out in other directions, from a painful area? (Draw on sketches.)
    - a. across the back
    - b. up the back
    - c. into the bottom
    - d. down the leg
      - (1) How far down the leg does pain go? (Draw on sketch.)
      - (2) Which leg? (Draw on sketch — front and back.)
11. When does your back hurt the most?   work-related? __
    - a. lying in bed __
    - b. driving __   after how long? _____
    - c. sitting __   after how long? _____
    - d. standing __   after how long? _____
    - e. bending __   after how long? _____
    - f. lifting __
      If lifting, from where: floor? __
                               table? __
                               crib? __
                               other? _____

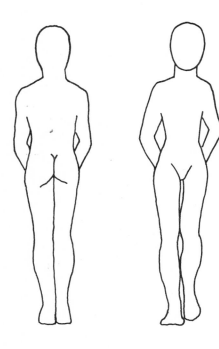

g. carrying __   after how long? _____
h. twisting __
i. other? Be specific. _____
12. Does the pain stop?
    a. For how long? _____
    b. When? under what circumstances? _____
    c. When does it start again? _____
    d. What eases it? _____
13. Have you had treatment? __   If so, what kind:
    a. exercises __   which ones? _____
        helped? __   how long? _____
    b. bed rest __   how long? _____
                      helped? __
    c. drugs __   which drugs? _____
                    taking them now? __   helped? __
                    how long? _____
    d. back brace __ how long? _____
                      helped? __
    e. traction __   how long? _____
        helped? __   how recently? _____
    f. surgery __   how many times? _____
                      helped? __
14. Has surgery been suggested if you haven't had it? __
15. Do you have lordosis (swayback)? __
16. Do you have back spasms (sudden cramps in muscles)?__
17. Do you have a short leg? __   Which one? _____
18. Is one hip higher than the other? __
19. Do you have scoliosis (side-to-side curve)? __   To which
    side at shoulder level? _____
20. Does constipation make your low back pain worse? __
21. Does a full bowel make it worse? __
22. Does menstruation make it worse? __
    a. how many days before? _____
    b. how long during? _____
An extra comments you feel might be helpful to complete
the information about your individual low back problem?

*This questionnaire would be useful to take to your doctor or
therapist to help remind you of all your symptoms.*

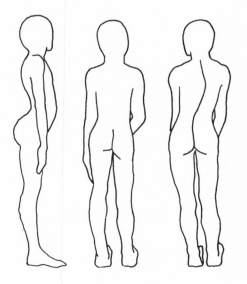

WHY YOU SHOULD SEE A DOCTOR

Without a diagnosis, you may never know what is causing your back pain.

> You may have a disease that's affecting your back.
>
> You may have an infection in some other part of your body that is giving you a referred pain.
>
> The bone may be degenerating.
>
> The disc may be degenerating or under compression.
>
> The cause may be simply a muscle in spasm.
>
> It may be a tear or pull of muscle or ligament.
>
> It may be a curvature of the spine.

The doctor should be a neurologist — time enough later to see a neuro*surgeon* or an orthopedist, if you need one. Most people do *not* need surgery for their low back problems; they need simple exercise of the right sort. All people should try long-term conservative treatment before considering surgery.

If you are told that you need surgery, get an independent opinion from a second doctor, who is, preferably, not a surgeon. He should not be associated with the first doctor.

If there is a difference of opinion, follow the most conservative methods of treatment suggested and, if possible, try to get a third opinion.

SOME PROBLEMS THAT MAY LEAD TO PAIN

Bone — misshapen, worn; fractured, slipped out of place; facets wearing on each other.

Disc — compressed; dried, shallow; ruptured, degenerating.

Muscles — tight where they should be loose; loose where they should be tight.

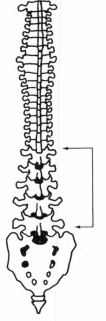

All vertebrae, as seen from behind.

five lumbar vertebrae

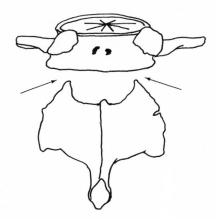

Fractured vertebra

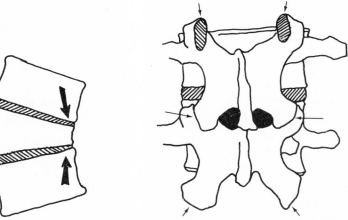

Misshapen, worn vertebrae

Facets — places where vertebrae glide on each other. Tissue wears away and region becomes painful.

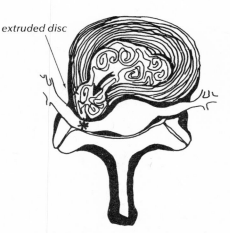

extruded disc

Looking down from above on one vertebra and its disc.

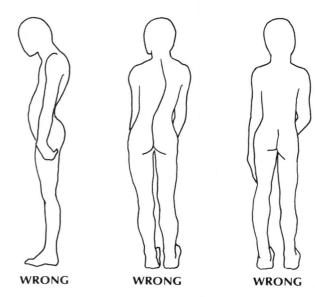

WRONG   **WRONG**   **WRONG**

Posture — round shoulders or swayback; side-to-side curve; uneven hips or one short leg.

Movement — limping; falling; jumping; opening windows incorrectly.

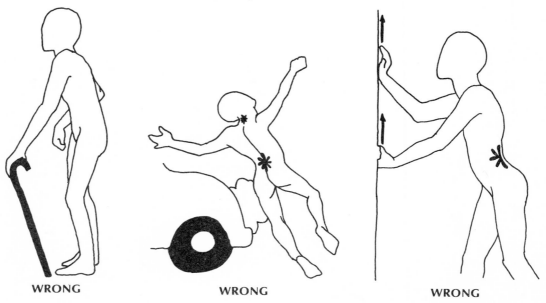

WRONG   **WRONG**   **WRONG**

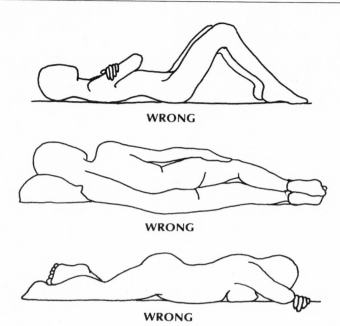

WRONG

WRONG

WRONG

Sleeping — tilting pelvis backwards; using sagging bed; lying on belly.

Lifting — bending from the waist; lifting with twist.

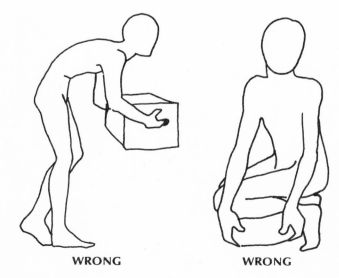

WRONG   **WRONG**

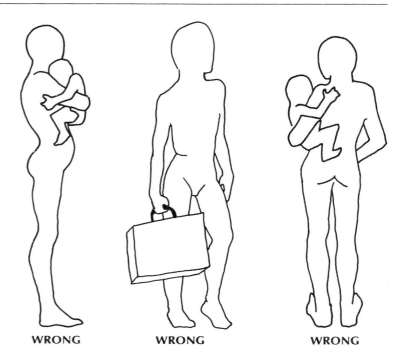

WRONG　　　　WRONG　　　　WRONG

Carrying — weight in front; one-sided lean; resting weight on one hip.
Sitting — upright sitting; legs too straight or seat too low.

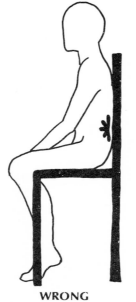

WRONG

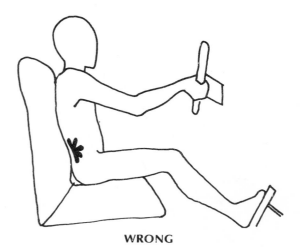

WRONG

Weather — chill; rain; cold; sudden change to cold; drafts; slippery weather.

Clothing — high heels; platform soles; constant use of girdles.

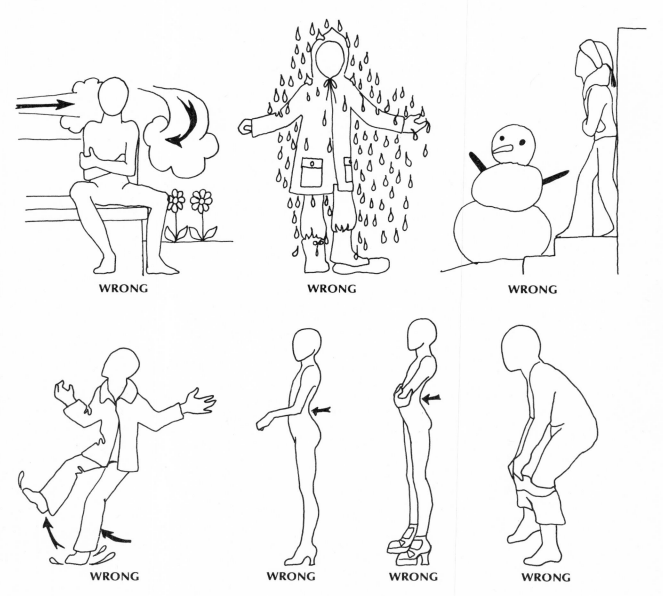

WRONG   WRONG   WRONG

WRONG   WRONG   WRONG   WRONG

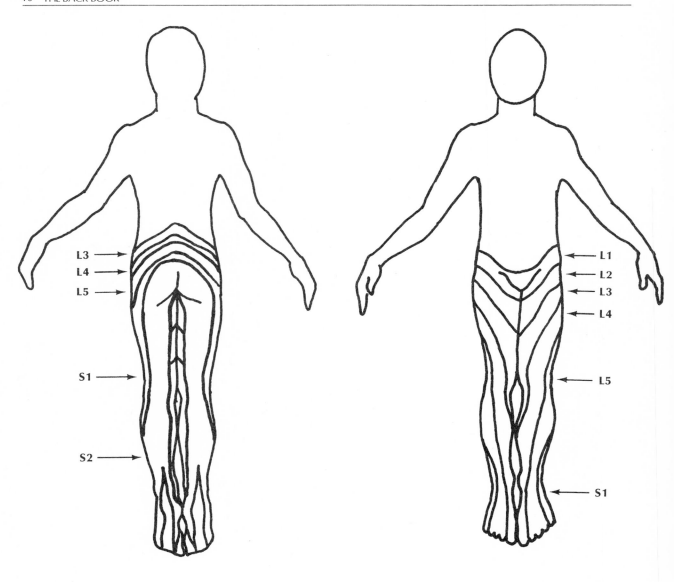

If you have pain, numbness, or tingling in one of these areas, the pain may indicate which lumbar segment is in trouble.

PAIN–TIME CHARTS

The following charts are to help you recognize those times when you do have pain, and try to detect what the possible causes could be. We shall then suggest ways in which you may alleviate the pain.

The questionnaire, along with the completed Pain–Time Charts, will give you a lot of information from which you can work by yourself, if your doctor has decided that improving the condition of your back is simply a matter of time and exercise.

When you do go to your doctor, it will help him if you take the questionnaire and all the Pain–Time Charts with you. Most of us tend to forget some small but important matter having to do with our pain as soon as we get into the doctor's office, or else it gets better momentarily and we may not remember where it was.

IMPORTANT There are seven identical charts in this chapter, one for each day of the week. Fill them in conscientiously; they will, when completed, present you with an invaluable picture of your own back pain and give you the basis for using the rest of this book.

The Pain–Time Charts will tell you:
   where the pain is coming from;
   where it extends to;
   maybe what's causing it;
   how often it occurs and how long it lasts;
   how you may be able to ease it;
   some possible ways to avoid it.

Pain-Time Chart

Name _____   Date _____

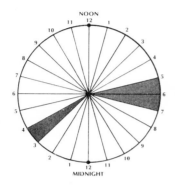

Pain?

When?

(Fill in times when
you hurt.)

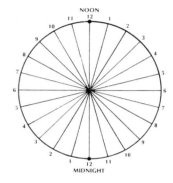

EXAMPLE

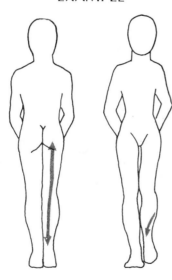

Pain?

Where?

(Draw arrows to cover
area that hurts.)

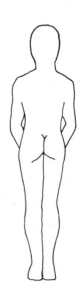 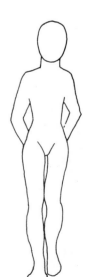

On the next page, fill in all information about the pain you
experienced for the rest of the day in case it either changed
in intensity, extended further, or became more localized.

Check proper squares — Fill in spaces

                                 Mins.   Hrs.   Days

How long ago did you last feel pain? _____
Was the pain: sharp? __ dull? __ intermittent? __ steady? __
Were you: standing? __   sitting? __   lying down? __

                    other   _____ _____

Were you wearing: high heels? __ flat shoes? __ lowered
                    heels? __ no footwear? __ girdle or
                    brace? __

How long ago did you last feel pain? _____
Was the pain: sharp? __ dull? __ intermittent? __ steady? __
Were you: standing? __   sitting? __   lying down? __

                    other   _____

Were you wearing: high heels? __ flat shoes? __ lowered
                    heels? __ no footwear? __ girdle or
                    brace? __

    Please try to fill in all the above information for *each time*
you have any low back pain.

Pain-Time Chart

Name _____ Date _____

Pain?

When?

(Fill in times when
you hurt.)

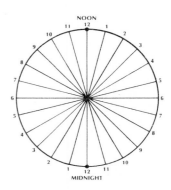

Pain?

Where?

(Draw arrows to cover
area that hurts.)

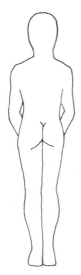

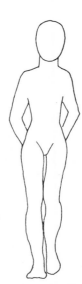

On the next page, fill in all information about the pain you
experienced for the rest of the day in case it either changed
in intensity, extended further, or became more localized.

Check proper squares — Fill in spaces

                                Mins. Hrs. Days

How long ago did you last feel pain? _____

Was the pain: sharp? __ dull? __ intermittent? __ steady? __

Were you: standing? __ sitting? __ lying down? __

                 other _____

Were you wearing: high heels? __ flat shoes? __ lowered heels? __ no footwear? __ girdle or brace? __

How long ago did you last feel pain? _____

Was the pain: sharp? __ dull? __ intermittent? __ steady? __

Were you: standing? __ sitting? __ lying down? __

                 other _____

Were you wearing: high heels? __ flat shoes? __ lowered heels? __ no footwear? __ girdle or brace? __

    Please try to fill in all the above information for *each time* you have any low back pain.

Pain·Time Chart

Name _____ Date _____

Pain?

When?

(Fill in times when
you hurt.)

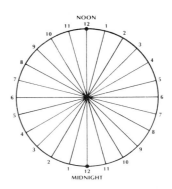

Pain?

Where?

(Draw arrows to cover
area that hurts.)

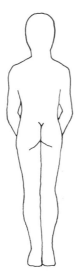

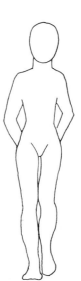

On the next page, fill in all information about the pain you
experienced for the rest of the day in case it either changed
in intensity, extended further, or became more localized.

Check proper squares — Fill in spaces

Mins.   Hrs.   Days

How long ago did you last feel pain? _____
Was the pain: sharp? __ dull? __ intermittent? __ steady? __
Were you: standing? __   sitting? __   lying down? __

other _____

Were you wearing: high heels? __ flat shoes? __ lowered
heels? __ no footwear? __ girdle or
brace? __

How long ago did you last feel pain? _____
Was the pain: sharp? __ dull? __ intermittent? __ steady? __
Were you: standing? __   sitting? __   lying down? __

other _____

Were you wearing: high heels? __ flat shoes? __ lowered
heels? __ no footwear? __ girdle or
brace? __

Please try to fill in all the above information for *each time*
you have any low back pain.

Pain·Time Chart

Name _____   Date _____

Pain?

When?

(Fill in times when
you hurt.)

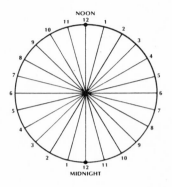

Pain?

Where?

(Draw arrows to cover
area that hurts.)

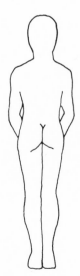

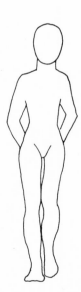

On the next page, fill in all information about the pain you
experienced for the rest of the day in case it either changed
in intensity, extended further, or became more localized.

Check proper squares — Fill in spaces

Mins. Hrs. Days

How long ago did you last feel pain? _____

Was the pain: sharp? __ dull? __ intermittent? __ steady? __

Were you: standing? __ sitting? __ lying down? __

                other _____

Were you wearing: high heels? __ flat shoes? __ lowered heels? __ no footwear? __ girdle or brace? __

How long ago did you last feel pain? _____

Was the pain: sharp? __ dull? __ intermittent? __ steady? __

Were you: standing? __ sitting? __ lying down? __

                other _____

Were you wearing: high heels? __ flat shoes? __ lowered heels? __ no footwear? __ girdle or brace? __

   Please try to fill in all the above information for *each time* you have any low back pain.

Pain-Time Chart

Name _____ Date _____

Pain?

When?

(Fill in times when
you hurt.)

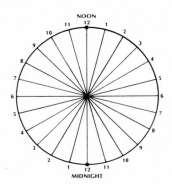

Pain?

Where?

(Draw arrows to cover
area that hurts.)

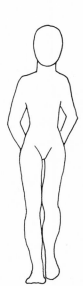

On the next page, fill in all information about the pain you
experienced for the rest of the day in case it either changed
in intensity, extended further, or became more localized.

Check proper squares — Fill in spaces

Mins.   Hrs.   Days

How long ago did you last feel pain? _____
Was the pain: sharp? __ dull? __ intermittent? __ steady? __
Were you: standing? __ sitting? __ lying down? __

other _____

Were you wearing: high heels? __ flat shoes? __ lowered
heels? __ no footwear? __ girdle or
brace? __

How long ago did you last feel pain? _____
Was the pain: sharp? __ dull? __ intermittent? __ steady? __
Were you: standing? __ sitting? __ lying down? __

other _____

Were you wearing: high heels? __ flat shoes? __ lowered
heels? __ no footwear? __ girdle or
brace? __

Please try to fill in all the above information for *each time*
you have any low back pain.

Pain·Time Chart

Name _____   Date _____

Pain?

When?

(Fill in times when
you hurt.)

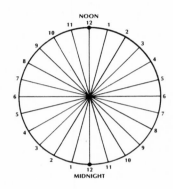

Pain?

Where?

(Draw arrows to cover
area that hurts.)

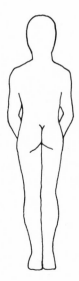

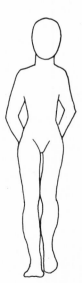

On the next page, fill in all information about the pain you
experienced for the rest of the day in case it either changed
in intensity, extended further, or became more localized.

Check proper squares — Fill in spaces

Mins. Hrs. Days

How long ago did you last feel pain? _____

Was the pain: sharp? __ dull? __ intermittent? __ steady? __

Were you: standing? __ sitting? __ lying down? __

           other _____

Were you wearing: high heels? __ flat shoes? __ lowered heels? __ no footwear? __ girdle or brace? __

How long ago did you last feel pain? _____

Was the pain: sharp? __ dull? __ intermittent? __ steady? __

Were you: standing? __ sitting? __ lying down? __

           other _____

Were you wearing: high heels? __ flat shoes? __ lowered heels? __ no footwear? __ girdle or brace? __

    Please try to fill in all the above information for *each time* you have any low back pain.

Pain-Time Chart

Name _____   Date _____

Pain?

When?

(Fill in times when
you hurt.)

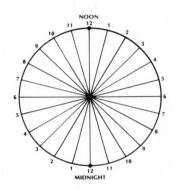

Pain?

Where?

(Draw arrows to cover
area that hurts.)

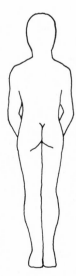

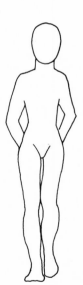

On the next page, fill in all information about the pain you
experienced for the rest of the day in case it either changed
in intensity, extended further, or became more localized.

Check proper squares — Fill in spaces

                              Mins.   Hrs.   Days

How long ago did you last feel pain? _____
Was the pain: sharp? __ dull? __ intermittent? __ steady? __
Were you: standing? __   sitting? __   lying down? __

                     other _____

Were you wearing: high heels? __ flat shoes? __ lowered
                  heels? __ no footwear? __ girdle or
                  brace? __

How long ago did you last feel pain? _____
Was the pain: sharp? __ dull? __ intermittent? __ steady? __
Were you: standing? __   sitting? __   lying down? __

                     other _____

Were you wearing: high heels? __ flat shoes? __ lowered
                  heels? __ no footwear? __ girdle or
                  brace? __

   Please try to fill in all the above information for *each time*
you have any low back pain.

Pain-Time Chart

Name _____   Date _____

Pain?

When?

(Fill in times when
you hurt.)

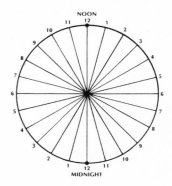

Pain?

Where?

(Draw arrows to cover
area that hurts.)

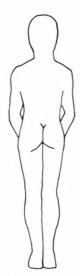

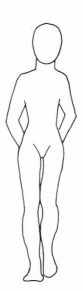

On the next page, fill in all information about the pain you
experienced for the rest of the day in case it either changed
in intensity, extended further, or became more localized.

Check proper squares — Fill in spaces

                              Mins.   Hrs.   Days

How long ago did you last feel pain? _____
Was the pain: sharp? __ dull? __ intermittent? __ steady? __
Were you: standing? __   sitting? __   lying down? __

                    other   _____

Were you wearing: high heels? __ flat shoes? __ lowered
                    heels? __ no footwear? __ girdle or
                    brace? __

How long ago did you last feel pain? _____
Was the pain: sharp? __ dull? __ intermittent? __ steady? __
Were you: standing? __   sitting? __   lying down? __

                    other   _____

Were you wearing: high heels? __ flat shoes? __ lowered
                    heels? __ no footwear? __ girdle or
                    brace? __

Please try to fill in all the above information for *each time*
you have any low back pain.

Look at your Pain–Time Charts. Is there any time that your back is free of pain?

Intermittent relief from low back pain means you almost certainly can prevent yourself from having low back pain again!

THE IMPORTANCE OF NOT CAUSING FURTHER BACK PAIN

IMPORTANT **As you continue, do not do anything (change position or posture, or exercise) that causes you pain. You will be inflaming, irritating, destroying, more tissue!**

Pain, whether sharp, dull, or intermittent, should not be allowed to continue. Your mission is to reduce the pain as promptly as possible, once you have become aware of it. Failure to do so will mean that more tissue will become involved and your pain will become more difficult to diminish or stop completely.

Pain is a danger signal. Do not ignore it. Recognize it and deal with it immediately. Discuss with your doctor whether you should cover it up completely with painkillers.

Watch out! There are some of you who will have become attached to that ache and will allow it as a constant companion! The luxury of staying ill, of being pitied, of being cared for, is frightening. Guard against it.

TWO

Options in Painkillers

PAINKILLERS

Please discuss this matter with your doctor!

You may very well have had painkillers prescribed if your back has kept you in constant pain. Low-level pains and aches can, in some cases, be completely hidden by such drugs, and you may find yourself making moves that you would not make if your back were still hurting. *Is this wise?*

For example, if poor standing posture causes you pain, should you change your posture instead of taking painkillers? If a poor sleeping position causes you pain, should you kill the pain with drugs, or should you consider the pain a warning that you're doing something wrong, and look for a change in sleeping position that may help ease your pain? If leaning against a sink or brushing your teeth causes low back pain, maybe you should think about changing the way you stand instead of taking painkillers.

IMPORTANT   Every one of the problems mentioned above can be bettered with proper positioning or proper posture.
   Is the theory worth testing?
   Are the painkillers curing you?
   Is your back getting better?

29

Maybe you could just dull the pain a little. Leave at least enough to serve as a signal so that you can develop ways to remedy the problem. It is an option worth discussing with your doctor!

Diazepam (Valium)

The compound diazepam, under the trade name of Valium, is probably the most commonly prescribed drug for low back pain, especially when the pain is accompanied by tension and anxiety. It is both a muscle-tone relaxant and a tranquilizer. But we seldom remember the warning by the doctor about its side effects, perhaps because we seek rapid relief. An information sheet comes with the manufacturer's package. But it is written in technical, medical language and the sheet is not always available to us with the repackaged prescription.

Every drug has side effects. But these effects are often so rare or so mild that, unless we are sensitive to the drug, we do not worry about them.

Diazepam is a different matter. It certainly reduces alertness. Driving under its influence is like driving with alcohol in you. And if you are working with machine tools, you can make dangerous mistakes. The compound heightens the effects of alcohol and barbiturates, so, if it is taken with a few beers or a sleeping pill, it will make you unusually drunk or sleepy. Furthermore, if you have been taking the drug steadily and heavily and suddenly stop, you may have withdrawal symptoms, just as with barbiturates or alcohol. These symptoms range from convulsions, cramps, vomiting, and sweating down to just plain nervousness and craving for "the hair of the dog that bit you" — more diazepam!

As is true of alcohol and barbiturates, Valium can even increase your problems. For example, you all know people whose anxiety is well controlled when they are sober, but who break down with a few drinks. The same can occur with this drug.

You all know people who tremble, and whose tremors become greater when they have had a few drinks. The same can occur with this drug.

There are people who are clumsy and whose clumsiness

gets worse with a few drinks. The same can occur with this drug.

The list is long.

But it is another matter, and perhaps a more worrisome one, that any drug that worsens your judgment makes it hard to judge for yourself how bad your judgment is (like the staggering drunk who insists that he can drive home — that he is quite competent). And you can become easily accommodated to your own bad judgment, attributing it to your nervousness, your pain, or your tension. This, of course, can form a vicious circle.

I have known many people who have been on this drug and later recalled how they felt under its influence and how they performed. Most of them were surprised on seeing the "warnings" insert that comes with the bottle. They had attributed their instability and uncertainty, their nervousness and tension, to their physical problem rather than to the treatment. ·

I am not urging you not to take the drug, but only to consider these factors if you do take it.

Investigation of any drug you consider taking is important to your well-being. Look at the insert that comes with the medication; if you do not find the insert, ask your pharmacist to supply one. Ask at your local library for the *Physician's Desk Reference (P.D.R.)* and, if there is none, ask the librarian to get one or to refer you to a place where you may read it. If you have trouble understanding the *P.D.R.*, discuss with your doctor the side effects of the drug you will be taking.

SPINAL FUSIONS

The enormous amount of freedom you have built into your structure has a lot to do with your many vertebrae. The soft material between each of the twenty-four bones of your back acts as a joint.

The one point where the movable vertebrae have a much more stable base — at the pelvis — is where most of us have our problems. The next two or three vertebrae above that location (the fifth, fourth, and third lumbar) take the largest share of the extra stress.

If you have enough pain and it continues for a long time, your doctor may decide that you would be better off with a fusion operation, which makes a rigid bridge at two points between two vertebrae to try to avoid the movement that is causing the pain.

The bridging of two vertebrae will automatically put more stress on the disc above and the disc below, but there will also be some extra stress on many of the other discs. You should, if you are considering such an operation, try to remember that some loss of flexibility should not just be expected, but should be designed into your future movements if you want to avoid more back problems. If your pain is leading you to think of taking any means to prevent further suffering, ask yourself first, "Have I really been patient in dealing with my day-to-day pain? Have I really done everything possible to prevent a recurrence of the painful episodes?"

You cannot undo a fusion operation. Convalescence can take anywhere from six to twenty-four months. With great patience and the right habits, more than three quarters of all people with low back pain can get rid of the pain without such surgery.

THREE

Easing Your Way Out of Pain- Position #1

When I am told about a magical gesture or a posture that is "best" for me, my intelligence rebels and I discount what I am told. In my experience, the more emphatic the teller, the less reliable the reason. Therefore I am a little, but only a little, embarrassed by insisting on a basic position for most people with low back pain.

It is precisely because there is so little freedom of movement in the lower back that the options are limited and it is possible to talk about a kind of optimum position for relaxing that region. So I will refer to this basic position, Position #1, over and over again as the primary step in easing pain.

What is Position #1? Lie on your side on a bed or sofa, with your knees slightly forward and bent, chin toward chest. This is called, when it is completed, the fetal position. It is modified, as will be explained, by pillows and small adjustments to relieve pain.

THE REASON FOR POSITION #1

A large number of people with low back problems suffer from extreme lordosis. There is a normal lordotic curve in

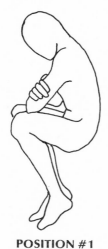

POSITION #1

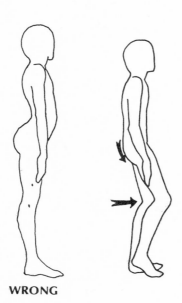

WRONG

the lower back, but when the few vertebrae directly above the pelvis begin to arch forward too far, an extreme lordosis is formed. Some arch is necessary to give your back a spring action. Too much arch defeats the purpose by taking the spring action to its limits, leaving no further spring action available to the spine when there is impact on it or weight added to it.

This one problem can cause pinching of the disc material; thinning of the disc material; extrusion of the disc material (the pushing out of some gluelike material from the disc, which can put pressure on a nerve); bulging of the disc wall, which also can put pressure on a nerve; breaking off of pieces of the vertebrae; rubbing together of parts of neighboring vertebrae; distortions of the vertebrae; swelling; and spasms.

All of these problems usually cause pain, sometimes severe, sometimes crippling.

Correct positioning is the most conservative treatment, with the best results, in the early treatment of severe low back pain.

Even when you are lying down, your pain can continue unless you position yourself in the proper way and unless you can train yourself to relax the tension that builds from pain and from spasms. It is important when your back hurts to try to relieve that pain.

Pain is a sign that damage is being done. That damage must be stopped first! Do as much as possible without causing yourself pain. It may take some time to let your back heal itself or to get into the habit of being free of pain, if the muscles undergoing small or large spasms, which are causing the pain, have to be stretched out. It may take some time to relieve the pressure of a disc bulging against the nerve. It will take some time just to train your lower back to achieve enough flexibility so that you eliminate the pain of one bony part rubbing against another, if that is what is happening. Certainly it takes some time to stretch the lower back muscles. It takes time to train the pelvis to greater flexibility so that it can be tucked under. It takes time to reposition the lower back so that a vertebra that has slipped forward can be positioned more comfortably over the pelvis.

IMPORTANT   Position #1 can give you the most freedom from pain for the longest period of time. If you use it wisely and at the proper time, it can, in many cases, completely free you of pain. Though this position may stop your pain, it will not solve your problem. It will prepare your body for the exercises that usually can solve your problem by making your back more flexible. Freedom from pain comes first!

BREATHING IN POSITION #1

There is a lot of tension that automatically occurs when you have pain in your lower back. On the other hand, if you have a chronic weakness in your lower back, everyday tensions can be enough to start a backache. It is hard to understand that you must positively — in a determined fashion — relax! But that is exactly what you must learn to do.

The whole of Position #1 is designed to relieve your lower back of all muscular pulls. There is no way this can be done unless you mean it to happen, help it to happen, and control the rate of speed at which it happens. This is how you do it.

With each small readjustment or easing of position in Position #1, close your eyes, inhale deeply (not so deeply that it hurts your back), and, as you exhale through your mouth, consciously but slowly and with control relax your back. If you relax too fast, it will hurt. Keep inhaling deeply and exhaling. The deep breathing alone will help you relax; each time you breath out, relax a little more. Keep your eyes closed and your mind's eye on your back muscles.

Tight shoulders, an arched neck, too rapid a change in position, can all keep your low back hurting. Check all possible points as you lie there and breathe in deeply — and breathe out — mouth open — eyes closed — and relax.

POSITIVE ASPECTS OF POSITIONING AND EXERCISING IN BED

If your back is in pain, it is very difficult to get down on the floor and back up without causing yourself more pain.

It is never necessary to get into any positions, or to do any exercises, on the floor!

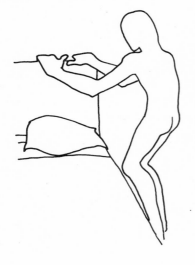

Position #1 is what you use when you are told to try "complete bed rest" for acute low back pain.

Position #1 is not an exercise! It is positioning, with many small easing adjustments, designed to help you free your back of pain.

HOW TO GET INTO BED

Since a good deal of your time must be spent in bed to relieve your pain, you need to know how to get into bed.

Stand with one side to the bed, knees slightly bent and your pelvis tucked tight under. Put your hand on the head- or footboard, or on the side of the bed, for support. Tighten your belly muscles!

Turning your back toward the bed, gently lower your bottom onto the bed, keeping your chin toward your chest.

Put your hands to one side on the bed. Roll yourself onto the bed sideways, bending your arms and putting less and less weight on your legs until, with knees bent, you can ease your legs onto the bed.

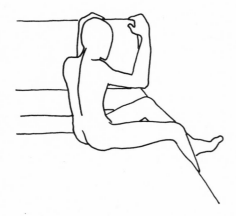

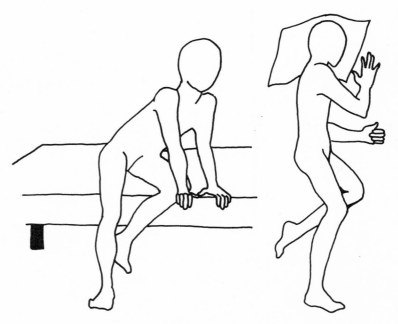

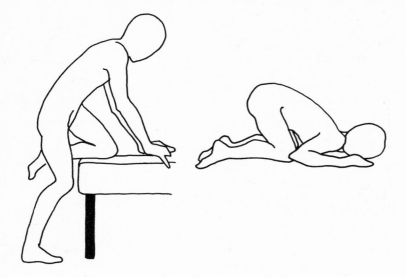

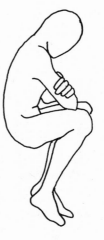

Alternate Method

Stand facing the bed, belly tight, bottom tucked under. As you lift one knee onto the bed, lower your hands to support yourself so that you can bring the other knee up. This will leave you in a kneeling position on the bed.

Crawl a little forward and then gently roll onto whichever side hurts the least.

WHICH SIDE TO LIE ON

Because of the nature of your individual low back problem, you may find that it is much easier for you to lie on one side of your body than the other.

Since the object of this entire project is to free you of pain, begin by spending a few minutes experimenting to find out which side is more comfortable for you to lie on.

Most of you will know immediately, because you have been forced by the pain to find out. Some of you will now become aware of the fact that you have, without being conscious of it, made a habit of lying on that side which causes you the least pain. Use the other side for variety. Roll back when pain begins.

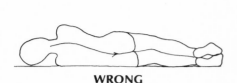

WRONG

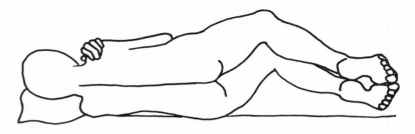

HOW TO USE A PILLOW UNDER YOUR HEAD

If you lie on your side without a pillow under your head, you will find that your spine at the neck has to bend to allow you to get your head to the bed.

Try to line up your spine so as to have it on one level horizontally.

Be sure that the pillow is not tucked under your shoulder. If it is a small or a very soft pillow, you may have to double it over.

Your nose must not be pointed either toward the floor or toward the ceiling, but straight ahead as you lie on your side. If the pillow is not wide enough to allow this, maybe a rolled-up blanket would be better.

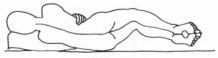

WRONG

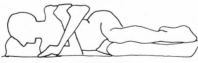

WRONG

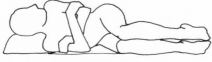

WRONG

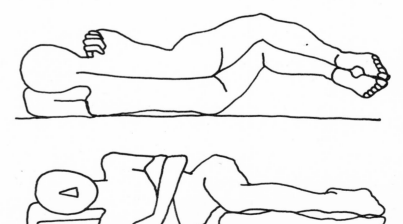

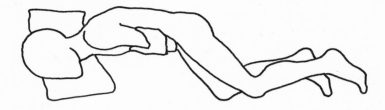

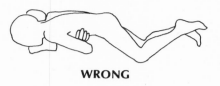

WRONG

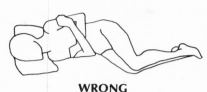

WRONG

Once your head is set, check your shoulders. *Your upper shoulder must be in a vertical line with your lower shoulder.* If it leans either forward or back, it will pull your spine out of alignment.

HOW TO USE A PILLOW BETWEEN YOUR LEGS

A pillow used between the knees or thighs will be good for some, bad for others. *You must judge for yourself.*

If you have a wide pelvis and thin legs, lying on your side will put a terrific strain on your upper hip joint and on your lower back. You must prevent your hip from being pulled over forward; it will drag on your lower back and cause more pain. One or two pillows between your knees or thighs — maybe a third between your ankles, or maybe even a rolled-up blanket — may be necessary to keep your knees in line with your hip joints.

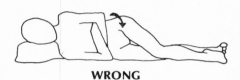

WRONG

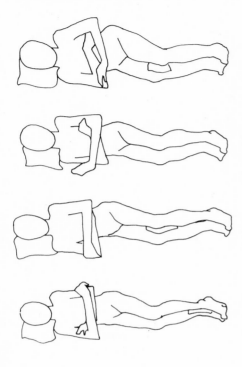

If your pelvis is wide but your legs are quite heavy, you may need only a small pillow between your knees, or none at all.

If your pelvis is narrow, most often you will not find it necessary to use a cushion or pillow between your thighs.

If your knees are bony or if you find that you have a tendency to let your hip tip toward the bed, put a folded towel between your knees. The folded towel will make you more comfortable if bony knees are your problem; if your upper hip tends to tilt forward or backward toward the bed, the towel will provide traction and will stabilize you.

You may even find that *bony ankles* cause you to position your legs in such a way as to pull your hip slightly off the position you need for comfort. Use a towel or pillow between your ankles also, if you need to.

PAIN IN POSITION #1

If your doctor tells you that you have an extruded disc, or if you have had low back surgery, or if pulling your knees up only as far as your hips gives you pain, try rounding your back in all the ways suggested in this whole section on Position #1.

Remain in that partly flexed position, chosen by you, that gives *you* the most relief from pain until the relief allows you to go further. *Do not hurry!*

You must not cause yourself more pain. Be patient!

SCIATIC PAIN

Sometimes sciatic pain increases in Position #1 when you are easing your knees to your chest or your chest to your knees.

If sciatic pain increases, stretch out a little that leg in which you feel the pain, until you reach the point where the pain eases. Each day, test to see whether the irritation has lessened enough for you to begin to ease in the leg that was more painful.

The leg that gives you no pain may be eased in as far as is comfortable. When one leg is in and the other leg is out, proper support for the upper leg changes. Use more pillows, if you must, to keep the *entire length* of your upper leg level with your hip.

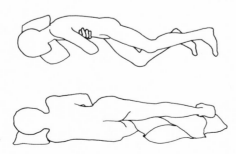

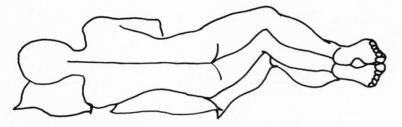

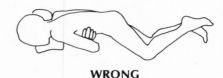

WRONG

HOW TO MAKE YOUR SPINE LEVEL ON THE BED

An important point to watch at all stages of Position #1 is the *distance of your spine from the bed*. Try to have a friend around to help you check it. You'll quickly learn the "feel" of a level back. Use as many pillows as necessary to keep all parts of your spine level.

A sagging spine can cause pain. Your shoulders must be in a vertical line and so must your hips!

Any shifting of your shoulders or hips, either forward or backward toward the bed, exerts a twisting action on your spine that will make you less comfortable.

Be sure to check your shoulders and hips often to maintain them upright. Rotating or twisting can cause you pain.

Narrow Waist

If you have an hourglass figure, you may find, while lying on your side, that your spine at the waistline dips way down toward the bed, leaving you with a lovely curve but an aching back.

Insert a folded towel under your waistline on the bed until, with a little experimenting, you find the right size or right number of folds in the towel to make you comfortable and to raise your spine to the horizontal.

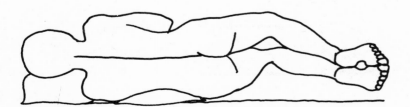

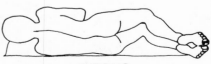

WRONG

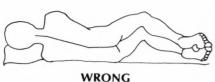

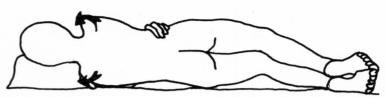

WRONG

Wide Shoulders

If your shoulders are wider than your hips, when you do get into Position #1 you are going to have your spine at an angle, with your shoulders higher than your hips. *This must be changed*.

If you can, roll or scrunch your shoulders forward evenly, so that your spine at the shoulders is lowered and your spine is then level all along its length. Check carefully to make sure that you are not twisting at any point along your spine. If you find it impossible to roll your shoulders forward, try folded blankets or a clean shag rug under your hips and legs to bring them to the right distance from the bed. This is just another way to line your spine up evenly.

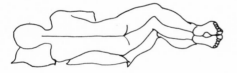

Narrow Shoulders

If you have narrow shoulders, the level of your spine through your hips will be higher than the level of your spine at your shoulders.

Wedge pillows under your shoulders and chest until your spine is an equal distance from the bed all the way along its length. Watch carefully that there are no twistings at any point along your spine.

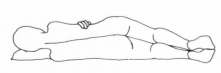
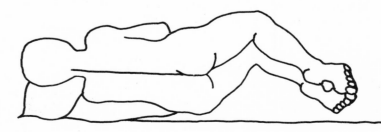

WRONG

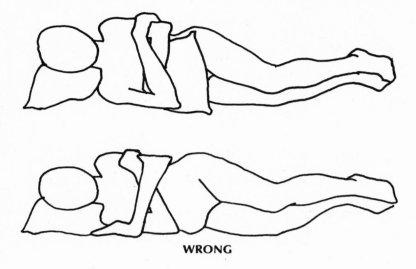

WRONG

FAKE BELLY-TIGHTENING

Quite often, sagging belly muscles can pull against the back even in Position #1. A pillow pulled tightly in against your belly sometimes will ease your back pain greatly.

EASING THIGHS TO CHEST

If this movement hurts at all, turn to page 46.

In a quiet room, where there will be no sudden movement, lie relaxed on the side of your body that is most comfortable for you.

Slide one hand *behind* each knee. If you put your hands in front of your knees and pull, you can stretch your knee ligaments. This is what you don't want to do. *Keep your hands behind your knees!*

IMPORTANT   Use movement that is so slow you can only feel it — not see it — to ease your knees very gently about a half-inch or less toward your chest. Pulling your knees in is too strong an action. E-a-s-e them in. If it feels right — just slightly taut — hold them right there. If it feels too tight or hurts at all, ease your knees out a little.

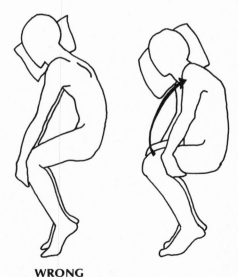

WRONG

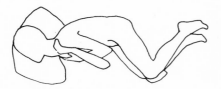

WRONG

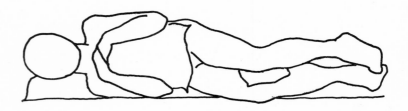

WHERE TO PUT YOUR ARMS

When you first get into Position #1, your arms should be in front of you. Your elbows should be bent, forearms crossed at the wrist (or where it is most comfortable for you), and your hands up under your chin. *Don't arch your head back!* Use another pillow between your arms if it makes you more comfortable.

As you bring your knees up or your head down far enough, this arm position becomes impossible. You can then just lift your arms in the same position up above your knees, or arrange yourself so that your arms are down along your legs, your elbows mostly unbent.

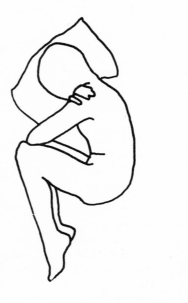
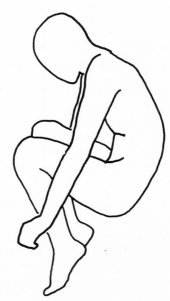

PROBLEMS OF OVERWEIGHT

When lying *on your side* in Position #1, try to arrange it, if you can, so that your knees are on either side of your belly, your belly lying between your thighs.

Ease your knees toward your *shoulders* instead of toward your chest. This gives you a better chance of getting your back into the proper curled position.

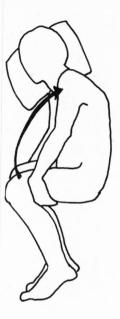

If the position above makes you feel breathless, try the sitting version of Position ;1 on a soft chair. (See page 129.) If this feels more comfortable, continue to use this position in the chair or on the sofa.

The sitting position puts more compression on the discs than the side-lying position. If it hurts, don't do it!

KEEPING SHOULDERS AND HIPS FROM TILTING

Slight discomfort may be felt if your hips or your shoulders tilt toward the bed. Check their position from time to time. Keep them from tilting forward or backward. Slight — very slight — shifts can make all the difference. *Move a little to reposition yourself for comfort, if it helps.*

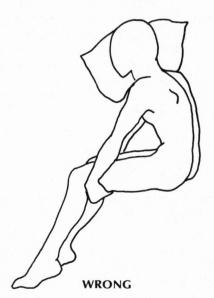

WRONG

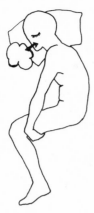

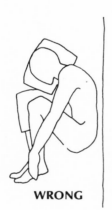

WRONG

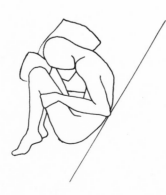

In this position, let your shoulders relax. Try it with your eyes closed. Inhale — and, as you exhale, *think about it consciously*; let your back relax!

Watch out! A sudden sharp pain may mean that you are relaxing too fast. *Relax slowly.* Ease the stretch out slowly. Continue to breathe and relax until your back feels completely comfortable.

When your back is relaxed, ease in your knees another half-inch, just until you feel a slight tautness in your back again. (The time between another half-inch easing-in can be minutes or days, according to your condition.)

HOW OFTEN TO USE POSITION #1

Try to get into this position every time you feel pain. If you are in constant pain and must work, get into this position *at least three times a day: morning, lunchtime, at night.*

The goal is to ease your knees in to your chest *with no pain*. Take whatever time your back needs (one hour to one month).

If you can finally reach the knee-to-chest position without having once felt pain and with only a slight increase of tension in your back as you moved your allotted half-inch closer, you have done well.

As you lie there, have someone else check you, if you can, to see if your waistline is the furthermost point on your back. If no one is there but you, lie in bed next to a wall, or on a sofa with a back, and check by feel that your waistline touches the wall or sofa and that your shoulders and hips do *not* touch the wall. Do not strain! Spend more time trying, gently and slowly, to ease more flexibility into your spine. If a large portion of your low back area still does not curve outwards, turn to page 65.

EASING CHIN TO CHEST

If the following movement hurts at all, turn to page 43. Try any of the other ways of getting into Position #1.

If you find that easing your chin down toward your chest is easier or more comfortable than easing your knees up, be sure to begin this way.

The very first move should be to tuck your chin into your chest *before* you begin to round your upper back.

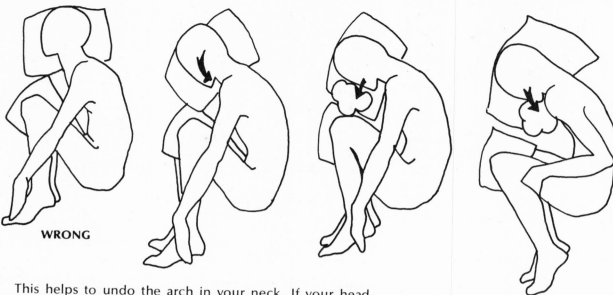

WRONG

This helps to undo the arch in your neck. If your head remains arched back, your neck and shoulder muscles, which need to be relaxed, will be tense.

Tuck your chin in first!

As you begin to tuck your chin in, inhale; as you exhale, let your chin ease in just a little further. *Don't let it hurt!*

Turn the front end of your pillow more toward your chest, to keep your chin supported. Then ease your chin *very gently* toward your chest, no more than a half-inch. Slip your hands behind your knees, if only to keep your knees from slipping down along the bed as your chin comes toward your chest.

If *this* position hurts, turn to page 50 or to pages 65–67. If it feels only a little tight, relax your neck as much as you can.

Ease your shoulders. Close your eyes, inhale, and, as you exhale (thinking about it consciously and feeling it), let your back relax. A sudden pain may mean that you're letting go too fast.

Relax gradually, slowly, gently, still in the same position. Check your shoulders and hips to see that they lean neither backward nor forward. Continue to inhale; exhale and relax your back at the same time — until your back and shoulders feel as relaxed as you can get them.

Never shift your position until you feel completely ready! Then ease your chin toward your chest another half-inch or less. If you feel that a half-inch is too much, ease it only enough to feel some slight tautness in your neck. Small shiftings can make you much more comfortable, but *stay in position!*

Your goal, the completed Position #1, is — *without any pain at all*, half-inch by half-inch — to get your chin to your chest; your chest toward your knees; the top of your head as close to your knees as possible; your back curled outward to make your waistline the furthermost point on your back.

Want to check it? Lie on a sofa or on a bed whose side is against a wall. When your waistline is touching the wall, your hips and shoulders should not be touching it!

If your chin is on your chest but your waistline is not the furthermost point on your back, turn to pages 65–67.

The easing-in itself is best done on an exhalation. Try it. Inhale. Now, as you exhale, let your chin relax further in toward your chest. Easier?

EASING IN FROM BOTH ENDS

If you can ease your chin gradually toward your chest and your knees gradually toward your chest without discomfort, try easing in from both ends.

First ease your chin in toward your chest, about a half-inch at a time. Then ease in your knees the same way. Use the careful methods laid out for chin-toward-chest, knees-toward-chest, alternately, as you continue working.

Inhale, and, as you exhale, let your back relax; close your eyes and *feel* it happen. If you run into any discomfort at all from easing either end, shift to easing just from one end for a while, until you can finally, *with no pain at any step*, get the top of your head as close to your knees as possible.

IMPORTANT   Do not speed up getting into Position #1 simply because your back is feeling better! This exercise or position is always to be done slowly and gently.

If you assume this position every night for your usual number of hours of sleep, you stand a pretty good chance of not having to assume it at all during the day.

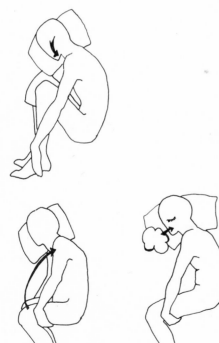

UNDOING TOUGH SPASMS

If you are lying in Position #1 with your knees easing toward your chest, your back spasms should begin to let up. If they do not, and the spasms occur in the area above your bottom and below your shoulders, there is a further step that you can take.

If the spasms are on your right side, lie on your left side; if the spasms are on your left side, lie on your right side. (For this explanation, we will assume that the spasms are on your right side.)

Lie on your left side. Ease your nose as close to your knees as possible. Slowly! No forcing!

This is the important next step: Fold a washcloth or a small towel and place it under your left side, right under the area that corresponds to the one on your right side where the spasms are occurring.

With a few adjustments, you should be able to place it just right so that it helps you to stretch out the muscles and undo your spasms more than you could manage by using only Position #1. Make sure that you use the breathing methods described throughout this section: inhale, and, as you exhale, concentrate on letting your whole back *relax*.

A small change . . . and it helps a lot!

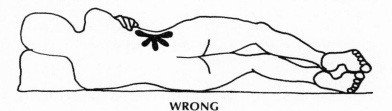

WRONG

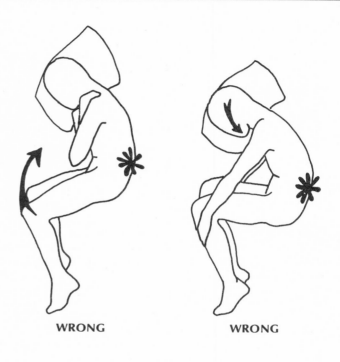

WRONG   **WRONG**

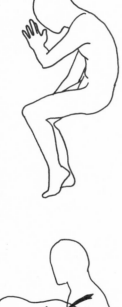

UNJAMMING TO EASE CHEST TOWARD KNEES

IMPORTANT   If you can't bring your knees toward your chest without pain, and if you can't bring your chin toward your chest without pain, you may find that you can bring your chest (your whole upper body) toward your knees with no pain at all! Try it gently to see.

Leave your knees where they are. Leave your chin up (but not arched back) and bring your whole upper torso forward. You'll need to use your hands on the bed to help you do this.

An extreme lordosis can "jam" some of the small bony projections of the vertebrae. Once your back is arched this much, pulling in from your chin or pulling up your knees may no longer serve to undo that arch. It may very likely be the cause of even more pain!

This is when easing your whole upper body forward may be necessary to undo the jam. To try to free your back up (to unjam it) from the direction of your pelvis, you must follow the directions on pages 65–67 and use pillows to accomplish, passively, the unjamming.

Quite often, after resting and easing in this position for a while, you may find that you can move your knees or your chin toward your chest without pain.

Try it. If it is still painful to do, relax — but continue to try at intervals to bring your upper torso forward.

Once the pain is eased by unjamming and irritation diminishes, the other easing moves can be begun again.

There is a very real difference between unjamming and overstretching. Proceed cautiously!

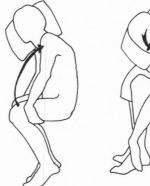
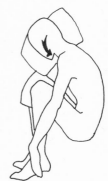

PAIN WHILE TRYING EASING POSITIONS

If you feel a real increase in pain while trying the easing positions, it may be that you are choosing the wrong adjustment for you. Check all the possible easing positions of Position #1. Try them to see if there is *even one* that you can use — one position that you can hold without increasing your pain.

IMPORTANT   If you have been in pain for a long time, if it looks as if you're going to have to live in pain, certainly it is better to get back on your feet and remain a part of the world!

You should let your doctor decide whether you can try the methods suggested in this book.

Few of us would choose to stay in bed just because of pain. If you and your doctor decide that you can and should keep trying, in spite of some pain, be sure you *never allow the pain to increase as you ease or shift in Position #1.* Stick close to your doctor's continuing advice.

IMPORTANT   An increase of pain is a signal that you are irritating tissue more. Our aim is to irritate it less. Reread the following each time you feel pain while holding easing positions.

Try again the different easing positions.
Ease into them more gently.
Hold each small shift in position longer than the last time.
Remember to use the breathing methods every time.

Whenever you feel pain in your lower back, get yourself into Position #1 *as soon as you possibly can.* If your work, or pain, prevents your getting into this position, check these position sketches for quick reminders. Find out how many will work for you.

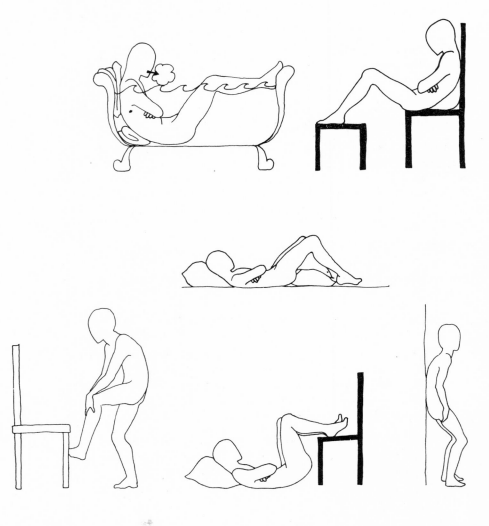

GETTING OUT OF POSITION #1

IMPORTANT   Don't move suddenly! Getting out of Position #1 must be as slow and gradual a process as getting into it. Otherwise, like a stretched rubber band suddenly released, the connective tissue will snap too far back, and you will feel pain.

Instead, *very slowly*, first just letting go of your knees with your hands, *gently* release all — even slight — tension. Now *slowly*, over a period of time, with your feet pointing toward the foot of the bed or sofa, let your knees ease out until, with your knees still bent enough to keep your lower back from moving, you can ease your legs over the edge of the bed to stand upright.

If that hurts, keep your knees against your chest (if, that is, they are already there!), roll over onto them, and then back slowly off the side of the bed, one leg at a time. Use the headboard to straighten up.

If you don't have a headboard on your bed, lean your hands on your knees. Tuck your pelvis under, tighten your belly muscles, and walk your hands up your thighs until you are standing.

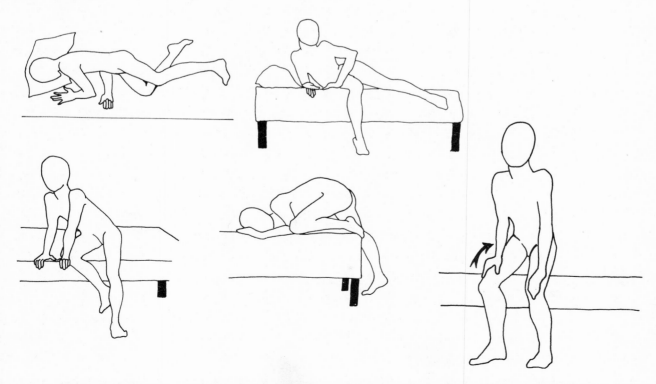

LYING STILL

The fluids in the disc become less fluid (like cold gelatin) with insufficient movement; ligaments contract slightly and muscle tone changes.

If you lie still for too long even in a good position, your back gets stiff and harder to move. It is good for you to begin small pain-free movements as soon as possible.

If you find yourself out of Position #1 during the night, but your back is not painful, there is no need to get back into Position #1 immediately. As time passes, this will probably happen more often. If your back begins to hurt, it will usually wake you. If it does wake you, then is the time to get back into Position #1.

Some varying of Position #1 should be what you aim for, once some of your pain is gone.

Movement is necessary to keep your back supple.

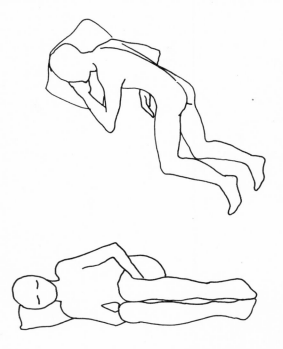

HOW LONG TO STAY
IN POSITION #1

Stay in the fetal position for one week — longer, if your pain dictates — making small adjustments for comfort.

Do not let the pain remain! Readjust slightly but immediately.

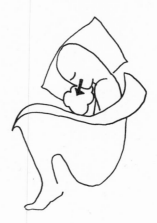

SLEEPING AND RESTING

At night, get into Position #1. Once your back is completely relaxed, or as relaxed as you can make it that day, use that position for sleeping. This gives you a head start on a pain-free night and will ease your back for the next day.

What if, in your sleep, you roll out of position? Curl back into it each time you find this has happened. *If you wake up in the morning out of position, take a while to ease yourself slowly back into the fetal position.* Think about your breathing. Inhale, and, while exhaling, concentrate with your eyes closed on letting your whole back relax. *Feel it relax.* This will ease your back and make getting up as pain-free as possible. Maybe even completely pain-free.

Any free moments during the day? Get back into Position #1. Make sure to use the breathing method described above. The more time you can keep your back free of pain, the less you are irritating the tissue and the sooner your back will be feeling better.

IMPORTANT   Like other unconsciously adopted tendencies, pain is a habit — a habit caused by poor position of your back or by pressure. Whatever the reason, you are the one who must break the habit!

The more often you can free your back of pain — the longer you can free yourself of pain — the less likely it is that the pain will return. Then, free of irritated tissue, you can begin to rebuild yourself in such a way as to prevent your back pain from returning.

Position #1 Check List

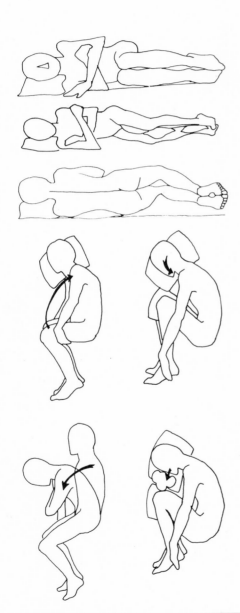

If you have really read and understood the preceding pages, you will never need them again. This page will give you a quick check list to use for positioning yourself for the night.

1. Lie on the side that gives you least pain. Bend your knees, with your arms in front of you.
2. Put a pillow under your head and point your nose straight ahead.
3. Put a pillow between your knees if you need it.
4. Put a pillow between your ankles if you need it.
5. Put a small pillow or towel under your waist if you need it.
6. Is your spine level?
7. Don't lift your head.
8. Don't twist.
9. Don't let your hips lean forward or backward (unless it eases your pain).
10. Don't let your shoulders lean forward or back (unless it eases your pain).
11. Use your hands behind your knees to ease them toward your chest — very slowly — as far as is comfortable (the easing-in should be so minute that it cannot be seen;
    — or ease your chin toward your chest;
    — or ease your whole upper body toward your knees.
12. **Be sure to close your eyes** (to help concentration); **inhale, and, as you exhale, relax your back completely.**
13. Since lying still produces some discomfort, **move slightly in ways that do not hurt. But maintain the basic fetal position.**
14. When you are ready to move out of Position #1, be sure to do it by slowly reversing those same movements you used to get into the position.

If your back kicks up, go back to the beginning of Position #1.

GETTING UP WHEN YOUR PAIN EASES

It is a beautiful relief to be free of pain after hours of suffering. Position #1, the fetal position, can give you that kind of relief. But it is a mistake to maintain that position for too long a period of time just because it gives you relief. Within a matter of days, you will lose a measurable amount of calcium from the vertebrae by not being on your feet. This leaves your vertebrae less capable of supporting you when you do get on your feet again.

IMPORTANT   While you are free of pain, try for at least a few minutes at a time to get up and walk around. Do not sit! Sitting will tend to cause you more pain! Lie down when your pain seems to be returning. Get back into Position #1! Do not wait for the pain to become full-blown. You can usually tell well in advance when the pain is about to hit again.

Refer to pages 75–79 for walking posture. A slightly exaggerated tucking under of your pelvis, a slightly exaggerated bending of your knees, will keep you free of pain a little longer when you are at this painful stage of recovery.

Sink stretches may help you to remain on your feet a little longer. See page 83.

IMPORTANT   Don't remain on your feet when your back begins to hurt again! Don't remain sitting in cars when your pain begins again! Lie down — on the car seat, on the floor (if a bed or sofa isn't handy) — but lie down! Get back in Position #1. Adjust the pillows. Breathe and relax the pain away.

USING THE PAIN–TIME CHART AS YOUR GUIDE

After you have kept a Pain–Time Study Sheet for seven days, you can begin to see a pattern; you can determine to some extent what is causing your back pain. You can tell just how many hours elapse between bouts of pain — when the pain starts; when it stops; what makes it worse or better. You can figure out from this information some ways in which you can eliminate some of your pain. Quite often you can get rid of simple problems *completely* with only one change of habit!

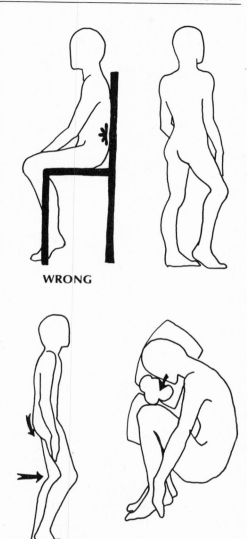

WRONG

Try this. Get into Position #1 *before* the pain gets to you. How? Look carefully at your Pain–Time Chart.

Do you have back pain *soon after going to bed*? Get into Position #1.

Do you *wake up in the morning* with back pain? It could simply be the result of the tightening of connective tissue as your body temperature drops while you sleep. Try wearing warm clothes; use a comforter or an electric blanket. Get into the habit of sleeping in Position #1.

Do you get back pain *after you've been up for an hour or two*? Figure the amount of time over a period of a week that you are free of pain before your back begins to hurt each morning. If you are up about two hours before your back begins to hurt, and it hurts more as the hours go by, it may be gravity that is causing the problem. Check your Pain–Time Chart and get into Position #1 about half an hour before your back is "scheduled" to hurt. After that, try to repeat Position #1 every few hours.

Is the pain *intermittent*? Check what you are doing when the pain begins. Check moves, positions, posture, clothing. Were you *sitting for a long period of time*? If you can learn to squat or lie down instead, you may be able to prevent the pain. If you work in a chair, get up often and ease your back. Try not to cross your legs. Try the Modified Position #1 for sitting. See pages 129–130.

Were you *standing still for a long period of time*? Get into the habit of shifting your weight from foot to foot.

Were you *wearing high heels*? Try wearing lower heels each day, if you can, until your shoes are flat.

Were you *leaning with your hips forward*? Learn to stand with your hips tucked under. If you're not strong enough yet to hold that position, put one foot up on a box or chair instead.

Were you *reaching for things high up overhead*? Try standing on a ladder to get things or put them in place.

Scoliosis Note

If you have scoliosis in addition to your low back pain, see page 108 for adjusting yourself in Position #1.

FOUR

Position #2

PROGRESS CHART

Now that you are free of some of your pain, you can begin the exercises that will hold you, finally, in a healthy standing position — one that you can easily maintain.

Fill in the following Progress Chart with the exercises that come after it. Make yourself more charts for the next few weeks to encourage yourself to gain strength and get into the right postural *habits*.

Marking on your chart your eight hours of sleeping in Position #1 will help give you a feeling of immediate success.

The Progress Chart will help you keep track of the number of periods you exercise and the amount of time you spend in a particular position. The left-hand square is for the sketch or description of one specific exercise or position. Fill in the times you do that exercise each day for a whole week, reading across the top of the page.

You may want to write in the number of times you did the exercise in one day;

  5 times
  4 times
  6 times

— or the amount of time you spent doing the exercise in one day;

  5 minutes
 15 minutes
 10 minutes

— or the actual time you began and finished the exercise in one day.

  8:00– 8:15 A.M.
 12:00–12:05 P.M.
  6:00– 6:30 P.M.

Use the method that is easiest for you. *Be sure to fill in the information for each time you exercise, each day. You chart your own success! Watch as you make yourself stronger!*

EXERCISE	MON	TUES	WED	THUR	FRI	SAT	SUN
#1							
#2							
#3							

PRECAUTIONS

Exercise simply means practice. When you are in pain, it is especially important that your position, your movement, your speed, and the number of repetitions of each exercise be under very careful control.

Without understanding and control, you cannot help yourself as well as you should be able to do. Please read and reread — slowly — as you perform each step — slowly!

When most of the pain is gone, it is time to get yourself gradually onto your feet. Your building program of positions and exercises can begin now. Passively protecting yourself from compression stress is important while you get the strength with which to protect yourself actively from compression. When you lie down, the discs are largely relieved of compression. There are fewer balance problems, and you can measure and arrange your posture to the bed surface.

IMPORTANT Although you may now be spending some time on your feet, all beginning positions and exercises must be done in bed!

CAUTIONS

The low back positions and movements that will be described in this chapter can be of great help to you if you use them as carefully as suggested. But remember: *No huffing! No puffing! No jerking! No bouncing! No hurrying! And no forcing!* Please use the information as it is meant to be used.

Among these beginning positions and movements you will find some that cause no pain. Which ones depends on your back problem. Try them all out at least once and, if necessary, start with *just one*.

Do only those exercises that do not hurt!

Your low back problem is just a little different from anyone else's. That difference is allowed for in this information.

All movement for low back pain must be slow, gentle, and persuasive if it is to help you gain new flexibility, new strength.

IMPORTANT   Trying to speed up the process by using force can only slow down your recovery!

In these movements, every action of yours creates a reaction in your back. You wouldn't yank on a dried-up, frayed rubber band, would you? You would stretch it carefully and gently, without too much repetition. The difference is that your back can change for the better — the rubber band cannot.

After using the comfortable positions and movements for two weeks, you may try again to do the ones that were painful for you in the beginning. Do *just one* of the suggested exercises that used to bother you. Slowly do that one exercise a few times — adding it to the ones you are already doing comfortably — *only if it doesn't hurt!* Wait until the next day to see if it has caused you any discomfort. If it has, discontinue it for now and wait for the pain to subside. Then try another of the suggested positions or movements and follow the same procedure. With the passage of time, you may be able to do most or all of them in perfect comfort!

INTRODUCING POSITION #2

Position #2 begins in bed, on your back with knees bent. Keeping your lower back flat on the bed, slowly extend your legs and arms with bottom and belly tight. This will finally become your new standing position.

If your knees are locked back when you are standing, your lower back goes into too great an arch. The farther back your knees are forced, the more your pelvis tilts and your lower back arches.

As your arms go up overhead, your back begins to arch more. The higher your arms go, the lower in your back the arch is forced. When your arms are completely extended overhead, your lower back may be quite arched. If you have any weakness in your lower back, you are in trouble in this position! Whether you can feel pain at the moment or not, your body is positioned, waiting for an accident to happen! Any push from behind, any object lifted up or taken down, and you are likely to be in pain.

The whole object of Position #2 is to strengthen you in just those ways that will protect you from these problems —

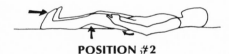

POSITION #2

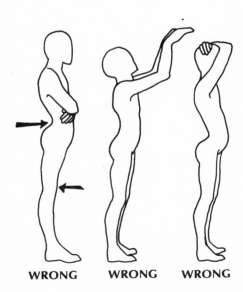

WRONG   WRONG   WRONG

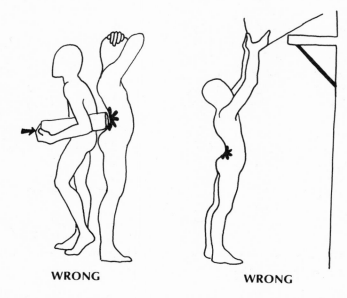

WRONG   **WRONG**

to give you the strength in standing, lifting, and carrying that, with continued practice, will protect you for a lifetime.

The exercise part of Position #2 is designed to make all the muscles of your bottom stronger. It is designed to strengthen all the muscles that rotate, or turn out, your legs. It works the muscles that extend, or straighten you out, at your hip and also works very well — beautifully — on your lower belly muscles. Once you have practiced it enough to know it well and to be able to hold the position for several minutes at a time (as long a period of time as you tend to spend standing), you then need do it only once a day in bed and, of course, change your habits of movement to make use of these same muscles constantly — every day!

Simple common sense will show you that the more often you repeat a movement that was initially unfamiliar, the sooner your body will recognize it and be able to repeat it on command.

IMPORTANT You must finally have enough strength to maintain yourself in a strong and safe standing position. The only way you will ever be sure that you can hold a position for, say, a half-hour or an hour is to build up till you can do just that.

If your muscles get tired as they try to hold you in a certain position, it is obvious that they are not strong enough — yet! It is necessary that you continue to hold specific muscles in contraction for longer and longer periods of time because you want *them* to hold *you* in position for longer and longer periods of time.

Before practicing the following stabilizing exercises, lie on your bed in such a position that you can feel the back of your waistline against the bed.

When your body tires, it tends to relax into using ligaments instead of muscles to stabilize you in an upright position. Your muscles become weaker and weaker from disuse; then the ligaments can become overworked, strained, and the cause of further problems.

Once you have gained the flexibility that comes with the practice of Position #1, practice Position #2 nightly until its daily use becomes a habit. It will help you to maintain yourself upright with the use of strong muscles.

ROLLING OVER IN BED

Lie down on, or turn onto, your most comfortable side. Then slip your hands behind your knees and *gently* ease your knees up toward your chest as far as they can go in comfort.

Keep your hands behind your knees and carefully roll onto your back, leaving your feet on the bed.

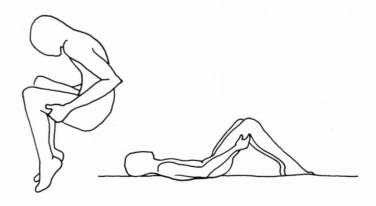

CHECK YOUR BACK FOR ARCHING

Before you start using Position #2, it is important to be sure that your back is able to maintain itself in a position that will guard against injury.

Lie on your back with your knees bent. Relax! Do not put a pillow under your head. In this position, and without effort, you should be able to ease the back of your waistline gently into the bed.

IMPORTANT Do not continue with the exercise portion of Position #2 until you can gently ease the back of your waistline into the bed!

Pressing the back of your waistline into the bed can be made easy if you put a pillow under your head or even put pillows under both your head and your bottom, as on pages 65–67. Go no further until you can keep the back of your waistline pressed against the bed!

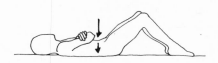

INITIAL FLEXIBILITY

Some people have lower backs that are so stiff — especially right at the waistline — that they cannot encourage their backs to straighten, let alone round out, even if they spend nights trying to sleep nose-to-knees.

IMPORTANT Force or jerking must never be used to try to encourage flexibility in a stiff or painful back!

Forceful or jerking movements can tear or irritate the tissue. The following is a trick that often helps people achieve flexibility.

Lie on your back, your feet on the bed, your knees bent. Ease a washcloth underneath your bottom and put a pillow underneath your head. Do this three or four times a day, maintaining the position for 5 minutes each time, or as long as you are comfortable.

In time — perhaps after several days — try a folded towel under your bottom in place of the washcloth. Use two pillows under your head instead of one, and later add another pillow under your shoulders. If the change causes you pain, increase the height under either end more gradually. Make smaller changes — hold each position for a few 5-minute intervals.

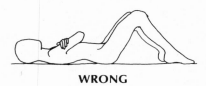

WRONG

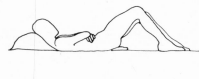

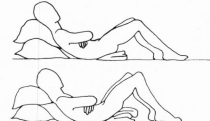

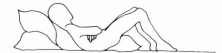

Again after the passage of some time, increase the thickness of the towel underneath your bottom, changing it finally for a pillow.

If you continue to get into this position day after day, the muscles in your lower back, the connective tissue in it, will slowly stretch into a more flexible and healthier condition and your spasms will be less frequent and severe.

IMPORTANT   If you have pain in your lower back and putting the towel or pillow under one end — say, your bottom — seems to cause even more pain, but putting the towel or pillow under the other end does not, listen to your body! Put the pillows under the end that does not hurt! Pain means irritation, and most often means further injury or swelling. Do not cause yourself pain. Make all changes gradually and with common sense!

BEGINNING TO BUILD YOUR BELLY STRENGTH

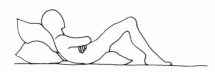

Get into Position #2 with pillows or something convenient and of the right size to elevate either one end or both ends of your body. Relax long enough for your waistline to ease toward the bed.

IMPORTANT   The breathing instructions change drastically from Position #1 to Position #2! In addition to relaxing your back, as you did in Position #1, you must tighten your belly. Be sure you make use of this change! It is very important to the position. The whole effect of the move is changed!

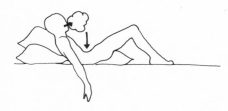

Inhale, and slowly, with your mouth *pursed* as you exhale, tighten your belly gently, and slowly ease and stretch your lower back down onto the surface of the bed. *Don't let go!* Just as slowly, inhale and let the stretch relax.

Now continue pursing your mouth to breathe out slowly as you continue to tighten your belly and stretch and ease your waistline onto the bed. Then inhale as you relax; continue inhaling and exhaling, stretching and relaxing, in a slow and rhythmic way.

This will help the part of your back that is the most inflexible — right at your waistline — to loosen up even further; you will have greater freedom of movement and can begin to develop some belly strength. That is what you will do as you breathe out. This belly strength will eventually help you to hold your back in a better position.

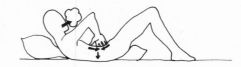

Want to know how to tell that you're building belly strength? Point all your fingers directly at your belly muscles. Push in a little. As you purse your mouth, breathe out and ease your back onto the bed. You should feel your belly muscles slowly tighten. That is the very beginning of the building of your belly strength. In this position, because the belly muscles are shortened, you are giving yourself an added bit of help. As you continue through different parts of Position #2, your belly muscles will become stronger and stronger.

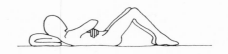

When you can, get your waistline to the bed and keep it there while you continue to breathe in and out normally. See if you can keep your waistline firmly fixed to the bed for one — two — five — ten minutes. In time, you should be able to keep it there as long as you like.

Now you're ready to move on to the next step.

IMPORTANT Do not ever press your feet or heels down in Position #2!

BEGINNING TO CLENCH OR TIGHTEN YOUR BOTTOM

When you have your *waistline flexible* enough so that you can keep it *tight to the bed* — when you can keep your *belly tight* and *breathe comfortably* while keeping it that way — then is the time to tighten your bottom.

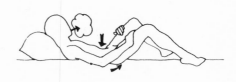

Turn your knees and feet out. Tighten your bottom slowly. Tighten it as hard as you can and keep it tight! *Don't do it over and over again!*

Tighten it and hold it tight!

As long as you can, continue to keep your bottom muscles tight (they will tend to relax). Do not pick up your bottom by pushing against the bed with your feet. Let the tight bottom muscles do the lifting.

IMPORTANT Don't relax your muscles or position! Retilt your pelvis! Retighten your belly! Reclench your bottom

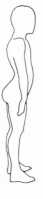

muscles until they tremble! Keep breathing! Hold this position each time as long as you can (each day you should be
able to hold the position longer, until you can hold it for at
least five minutes at a time. Release from this position very
slowly!

REMINDER   Never bear down with your feet or heels during Position #2!

PROBLEMS WITH A BIG BOTTOM

A large bottom will tend to swing your pelvis farther back
when you stand, causing you much discomfort and a very
arched lower back.

To offset this tendency, you will have to get the lower part
of your spine even more flexible than it need be in other
circumstances, and your bottom and lower belly muscles
extremely strong, in order to maintain the pelvis in the
proper position.

Go after the same easing-down of your spine to the bed as
was recommended for the usual swayback (see pages
65–67). It may take you a little longer, but the final position
of your pelvis will be worth it.

Once you can keep your lower spine against the bed,
move on to the rest of the steps in Position #2. They will
strengthen your pelvic support muscles so that you can
maintain something close to this posture when you are
standing on your feet.

Don't expect your bottom to get smaller, although, if the
muscles are loose to begin with, it may look smaller as the
muscles tighten.

SCIATIC PAIN

If you have sciatic pain, clenching your bottom muscles can
in some cases be painful. Be sure that you clench your bottom muscles very gently, very lightly, at first. Hold that position as long as you can. When you can't hold it any longer,
let your muscles relax just as gently as they were clenched.
Stop if you feel any pain when clenching!

During the first several days, do very few clenches and
give yourself time to see what the results are. If your sciatic

pain gets at all worse, the clenching should be done fewer times and even more gently. If you have no increase of pain, continue to increase gradually the amount of contraction you are putting into the muscles of your bottom.

If you have had sciatic pain, you don't need to be told that it can come on at odd times, and that sometimes it is really impossible to figure out what caused the pain. *Any time it hurts, go back to more gentle bottom clenchings for a while.* When the sciatic nerve is irritated, further irritation serves no good purpose. Work your way back gradually each time. If you are very good to yourself and continue your exercises faithfully, you may have little or no further pain.

PAIN CAUSED BY PILLOW

This is important to check.

If having your head on a pillow causes you real discomfort, you will want to do these exercises without a pillow. On the other hand, it is likely that if your belly muscles are weak, going without a pillow when you're doing the exercise (movement) will make you arch your head and neck. This pushes the top or back of your head into the bed, which makes you tense your shoulder muscles and also makes you tighten your back muscles instead of stretching them. It can cause you a lot of pain!

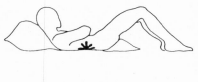

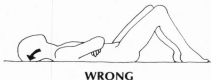

WRONG

Until you have created in your body a real awareness about which muscles should be tight, which stretched, it is best to elevate the head, if only a little — as long as it does not cause pain! If the elevation really does cause pain, try a smaller pillow. Or try a folded towel.

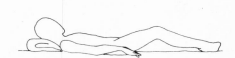

Your chin should always be tucked into your chest, to prevent your using any of the backward pressure that comes from pushing your head into the bed.

CONTINUING TO CLENCH OR TIGHTEN YOUR BOTTOM

Throughout this Position #2 exercise, you are slowly beginning, and continuing, to develop in a lying-down position the stretches and strengths that you need through the pelvic and abdominal girdle. These will help you finally to maintain

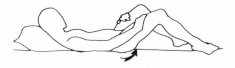

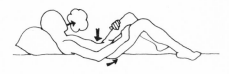

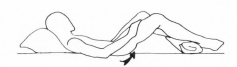

good posture when you are standing. Watch the way the position — and your body — develop as you go on!

Lie on your back with a pillow under your head, your knees bent, feet and knees turned out, your arms at your sides, and hands on your thighs. With your mouth pursed, breathe *out* as you slowly tighten *only* your bottom. Do it slowly, gently, but tighten your bottom as much as you can. At this stage, breathing out will help tighten your belly to force your waistline into the surface of the bed. Keep your hands on your thighs. Feel them as you tighten your bottom. Your thighs should not tighten! Your feet should not press into the bed. Put your ankles up on a rolled-up blanket — even on the seat of a chair, if you must — to prevent using pressure from your feet. *Only your bottom should tighten!* Hold that position as long as you can. Untighten your bottom *slowly* — just as slowly as you tightened it — while you inhale. Repeat slowly as often as you like until you gain some strength.

IMPORTANT   Breathe normally!

As you become stronger, keep your back forced down onto the surface of the bed, slowly tighten your bottom as hard as you can, and continue to hold it very tight *as you continue to breathe normally*. Hold it tight as long as you can — until your bottom trembles — then, still *breathing normally, very slowly* let your bottom relax. If you've really been holding your bottom tight, it may tremble its way unevenly into its looser state.

IMPORTANT   Pay close attention! Do not let yourself lift your bottom! Your back must not do any lifting! Your waistline must stay tightly pressed to the bed! Your feet must not do any pressing down!

The clenching muscles will eventually be strong enough to lift your pelvis and to hold it tight.

EXTENDING LEGS IN POSITION #2

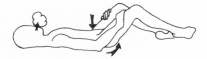

Once the preceding exercise becomes easy for you, and you are doing it about 25 times a day, shift to doing this one. If it causes any pain, go back to the former version.

Take the same Position #2, with your knees and feet turned out. Breathe normally. Keep your lower back tightly pressed to the bed. Tighten your bottom muscles *slowly and as hard as you can* — harder! Hold it! Relax slowly. Stretch your feet out a little farther along the surface. Stop them there. Then *slowly* tighten your bottom muscles again. Keep your waistline tight to the bed, your back flat, the entire time! Only your bottom muscles should relax and then tighten — the back of your waistline *stays down!* Breathe normally while you keep your belly tight, your waistline tight to the bed, and your bottom clenched.

Keep practicing this new position until the tightening of your bottom becomes easy for you, and until you can hold it as long as you like, with your waistline pressed right into the surface of the bed.

Move your feet along another few inches and start again. Keep repeating, stretching your feet farther along the bed each day or week as you are able. **No hurry! Too fast and you will lose the proper position!** Take it at the rate of speed that keeps you comfortable.

Finally stretch your legs out as straight as you can get them, with your feet turned out and your knees *slightly* bent, and still keep the back of your waistline down when you tighten your bottom. Keep practicing until you can finally tighten your bottom hard and press your waistline firmly into the bed and hold that position for many minutes while you breathe normally.

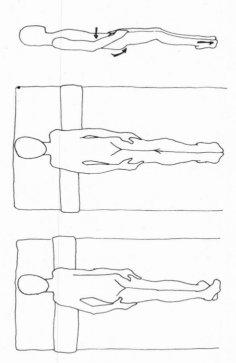

Your feet will tend to turn out more as you get them farther out along the bed. Work that way for a while. Next, try to keep your feet together — heels and big toes touching — as you tighten your bottom as hard as you can and keep your waistline close in to the bed.

It becomes useful as you work to *hold this position* over extended periods of time, using the muscles differently. Then cross one foot over the top of the other and use this added force to help you to tighten your bottom further, and again differently, and ease your knees closer to the bed. First cross your right foot over the left and tighten as hard as you can and hold that position; then cross your left foot over the right and again tighten as hard as you can and hold that position.

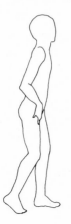

FOOT-POSITIONING FOR STANDING AND WALKING

When you finally do stand up, you will not just want to stand there! Before you get up, you should be able to bend your feet at the ankles up toward your knees, so that when you have to bend your feet for walking, you will be able to!

Still in Position #2, lie on your back with no pillow under your head. The back of your waistline should be pushed against the bed, your bottom should be as tight as possible, your feet turned out or straight, and your legs stretched out straight along the bed with knees only slightly bent.

Now add this step:

As you lie there with everything in the proper position, bend your feet at the ankle to bring the feet as far toward your knees as possible. Try both feet at once; very slowly and gently turn them up as far as is comfortable. Then try it with both feet pointed downward as far as possible (since you may want to walk downhill too). Continue to practice this movement until you can hold the position without discomfort for as long as you like.

Keep your waistline right on the bed the whole time! Keep your knees just slightly bent!

Now try pushing one foot down as the other comes up, both for variety and for developing the right rhythm for walking — especially if you have been off your feet for a long period of time.

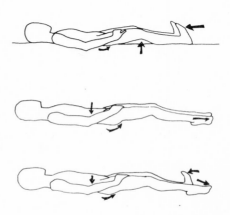

DEVELOPING POSTURE FOR OVERHEAD LIFTING

While in Position #2 on the bed, you must continue to develop, in this nice safe position, those abilities you will need when standing upright.

It is a fact that if you lift your arms overhead while you are standing, your back begins to arch as your arms go up. As your arms reach higher and higher, this arch in your back is carried farther and farther down; that arching causes an extreme lordosis.

You can learn to control the arch; you can straighten it somewhat, or you can prevent the arch by standing on a stepladder instead of reaching your arms overhead. Strengthening and controlling the arch is preferable.

This is the approach: Lie in the fully extended position (Position #2), with all of the proper muscles taut and your toes pointed (this time to simulate standing on your toes, which you often do when you must put something up high overhead). Since this position would normally cause your back to arch more if your were standing, you will, of course, prevent it from arching by forcing your waistline down into the bed! **Keep breathing in the normal way!**

Now add to the simulation by putting your arms behind your head. **Do not allow your back to arch!** Relax your position and tighten again as you need to. When it is easy to prevent your waistline from rising up from the bed in this new position, begin slowly to raise your arms along the bed farther above your head, developing strength at each point, until it is easy to keep your waistline tight to the bed without too much trouble. **Keep breathing!**

Continue until your arms are stretched straight up overhead and you are still able to keep your waistline tight to the bed, your bottom tight, your toes pointed, and your breathing normal.

You should now be able, when you are on your feet, to stretch up overhead, to put things away or take them down, with enough control so that you will not hurt yourself.

IMPORTANT Recognize that this is only a precaution! Weight from overhead will still compress your spinal column. When possible, try to use a stepladder to put things overhead or to bring them down.

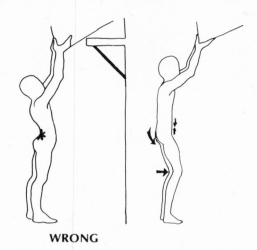

WRONG

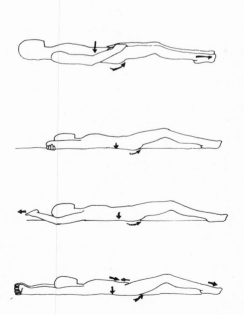

HIP FLEXIBILITY

The final step in Position #2 is also the one that should be continued on a *daily basis.* This will keep your back in excellent condition when used in conjunction with Position #1, Position #3, and several habits and tricks that need to be learned.

Lie in Position #2, one leg stretched out, your waistline eased onto the bed, your feet turned up at the ankles toward your knees, your bottom as tight as possible, and the knee of your extended leg eased down toward the bed — not locked back!

Tighten your belly muscles and bring one knee in toward your chest, *gently.* If you must, hold it there for a while with your hands behind your knee. Over a period of time, your own flexibility and strength should grow so that you can maintain knee-to-chest *without using your hands* while the rest of your body is in extended Position #2.

Hold it there. Keep your belly tight as you lower your leg to the bed. Then bring the other leg up and repeat the hold. Hold it as long as you can. Tighten your belly harder as you lower your leg to the bed when you're not holding on. Then do the same with your other knee.

Finally, try this exercise while you slowly extend your arms until they are completely stretched overhead. Hold this position as long as you can.

Breathe normally throughout the entire exercise.

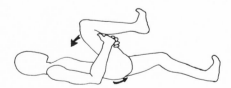

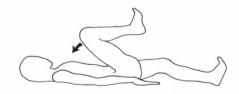

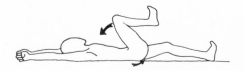

GETTING RID OF THE PILLOW

When you finally use this position in standing, there are some obvious points to be considered. You don't want your chin hanging forward, so get the pillow or towel out from underneath your head if you have not already done so.

Get into the same position as you do for Position #2. Remove the pillow from under your head, if you can, and still maintain your position with your waistline flat on the bed. If getting the pillow out all at once is too fast, try using a slightly smaller folded towel each day. Stop if you experience any pain, or if you begin to arch your head back.

Position #2 will strengthen the lower back in the proper position. It will also strengthen your bottom muscles and your outer thighs. These strengths will help you to maintain a position while standing that should help relieve much of your discomfort or pain.

HOW CAN YOU STAND THAT WAY?

Bending your knees when you stand places your pelvis easily in the best position to allow you to maintain the proper standing and walking positions. This position uses your thigh muscles, bottom muscles, long back and belly muscles.

How much should you bend your knees? Just enough so that they are slightly unlocked. When your belly muscles are overstretched from either locked knees or overstretched hip joints, they are extremely difficult to tighten.

As soon as your hips and knees are just very slightly flexed, the belly muscles — a little loosened from their overstretched position — can be tightened much more easily and much harder. Flexing your hips and knees slightly when you stand and walk makes it easy to tighten your belly muscles.

Tight belly muscles help to maintain you' in the upright position without undue pressure on lumbar discs.

Overstretched belly muscles prevent any tightening.
Leaning on hip ligaments stretches belly muscles.
Locked knees stretch the belly muscles.
Overweight stretches belly muscles.

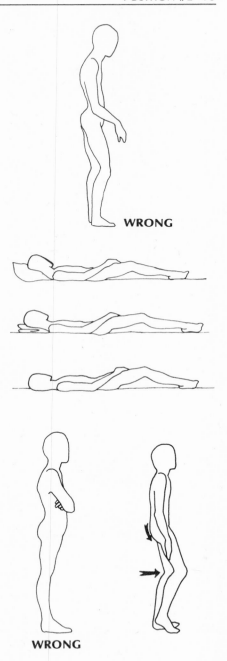

WRONG

WRONG

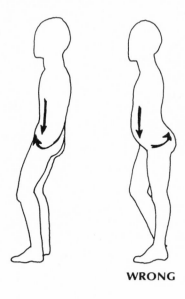

WRONG

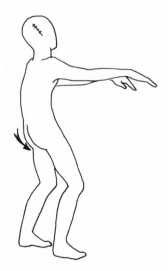

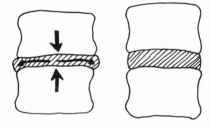

ON YOUR FEET AND WALKING

The bottom-tightening exercise that you do while lying down with your knees bent must eventually be done in a standing position, with your knees just unlocked, if you are going to be able to walk long distances without pain.

Your pelvis can be considered a basin, which, if tipped, will let its contents hang over the edge. So a slightly tipped pelvis can let your innards hang out and lean against the belly wall. You should try to tip it up in front so that it can better support your innards.

When you first begin trying to walk with your bottom tight, you may feel like a product of Baron Frankenstein's laboratory. Practice as long as your bottom-tightening can hold out! In time, the walking will ease, your bottom muscles will strengthen, and, with constant reminders to yourself, this position will become a habit. Then you will, at last, be able to maintain better posture and help relieve your back.

Between each bone, or vertebra, of your spine is a small balloonlike area, confined by heavy mesh and filled with a thick gluey substance that serves, in one sense, as a shock absorber. Walk in such a way as to prevent heavy pressure

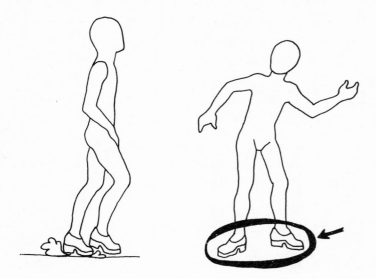

on these "balloons." A floating action rather than a bouncing action is what you should ease into. Bouncing is fine once you are free of pain and learn to use your arches, knees, hips, and spine. Maybe you have seen slow-motion pictures of a good gymnast on a trampoline. Start with conquering the "floating" action; your body will then automatically know how to bounce.

You should try to do all walking from this time forward with your bottom tight and your pelvis tucked under or up in front and with your knees just slightly bent, as in Position #2 on your bed. All the exercises on these pages, if they are adopted as habits, will minimize the chance of a recurrence of your back problems.

When walking:

1. Wear flat shoes with soft soles. This automatically improves your balance and posture and softens impact.
2. Turn your feet outward slightly to improve your balance. If fear of pain has you walking more slowly, take smaller steps and set your feet down a little farther apart.
3. Bend your knees (keep them just unlocked) to make you use your thigh muscles. This will help you to tuck your bottom under more easily.

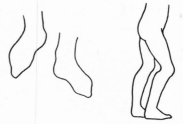

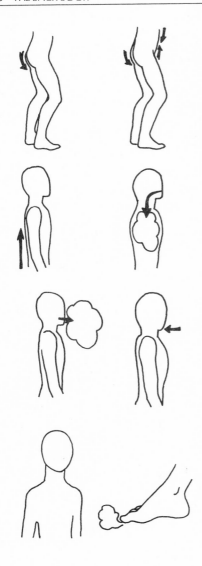

4. Tighten your bottom hard with each step — right side of your bottom when your right foot goes down; left side when the left foot goes down. This helps tuck your bottom under.
5. Tighten your lower belly muscles.
6. Lift your chest.
7. Inhale a little more than you usually do; exhale a little more than you usually do.
8. Keep your head up and your chin in a little.
9. Have your shoulders slightly down and loose so that they swing for balance.
10. Remember that the less noise your feet make as they come in contact with the floor, the less you are jarring your spine.

STANDING AND WALKING CAN HURT!

Extra pressure on your spine tends to cause more pain. Let's go into that a little.

When you have been up for several hours and on your feet or sitting down, the gravity that affects us all compresses the discs between your vertebrae, pressing them down so that by the end of the day you can be one-quarter to three-quarters of an inch shorter! The weight of the upper part of the body puts pressure on your lower back, squishes each disc down (the way you would put pressure on a balloon with a hand above and below), and, where there is tender or irritated tissue, causes you more pain or discomfort. You can undo this to some extent with the sink stretch (page 83) or the overhead stretch (page 88). If your back is terribly painful, Position #1 or its alternatives are best (pages 33–55).

This slight squeeze happens to all of us. Undo it as often as you can. If you wear hard-soled shoes, walk on hard pavements, walk by pushing your heel into the floor first, or make a thump as you walk, you are creating an impact that can only make your back hurt more. It is always important (but if you have a back problem, more important than ever!) to wear soft-soled shoes — thick, flat, soft soles — if you must walk on hard pavement. It is also important to learn to walk lightly, making as little noise as possible, and to learn to walk more toe-heel than heel-toe.

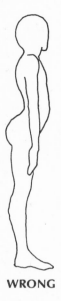

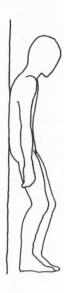

WRONG

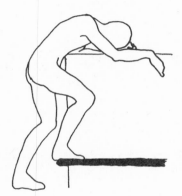

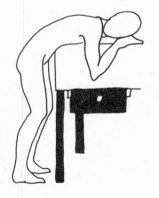

IMPORTANT   To prevent impact (fast compression of the spine) from being quite so severe, you must remember to keep your knees slightly bent at all times when you walk. Just unlocked — no need to carry it to Groucho Marx extremes! This allows you to use your knee as a shock absorber. Locking the back of the knee not only jars your body when you walk, but also forces your lower back into an extreme lordosis. An extreme lordosis is that curve-in above the bottom that you are working so hard to undo to stop your back from hurting.

When you're trapped in a place where you can only stand, try this. Back yourself up against a wall, with the back of your waistline touching the wall, and your feet a little way out. Tighten your belly muscles to take some of the stress off your lower back; then shift your feet around till you find the most comfortable way to place them to ease your back discomfort. As an alternative, try draping yourself over a piano — a bar, a counter — or anything that serves to relieve your pain. *Remember: Pain must not be allowed to continue.*

Position #2 Check List

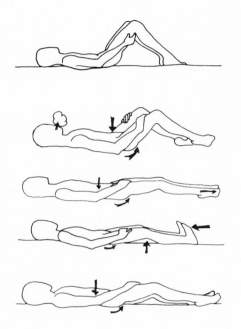

If you have read carefully and really understood all parts of Position #2 and have worked your way carefully through them, if you practice the move daily, you will never need the foregoing pages again. What follows is a quick check list, which you can use to remind yourself daily of the proper positioning, movements, and the ways in which you should hold the position.

1. Lie on your back slantwise on the bed; no pillow; knees bent.
2. Breathe out to tighten your belly and ease your back down to the bed.
3. **Keep your back down and belly tight, but begin breathing normally!**
4. Tighten your bottom hard and slide your legs out.
5. Keep your back tight to the bed, your belly tight, your bottom tight. Continue to breathe normally and pull the front of your feet up toward your knees.
6. With your back tight to the bed, your belly tight, hold this position as long as you can with your feet turned out.
7. Next, with your back tight to the bed and your belly tight, hold this position, breathing normally, with your feet together.

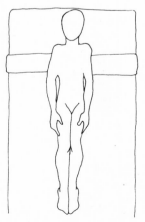

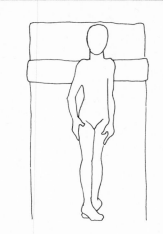

8. With the back of your waistline tight to the bed and your belly tight, breathe normally, your bottom tight, and hold this position, crossing one foot over the other — then the other foot over.

9. With the back of your waistline tight to the bed, breathe normally, holding your belly, bottom, legs, and feet hard and tight; move your arms high above your head.

10. **Keep the back of your waistline firmly down to the bed; continue to breathe normally, with your bottom and belly tight. Then stretch your legs and feet out firmly, stretch your arms out high overhead, and now, just like that, hold — as long as possible! Repeat two or three times each day.**

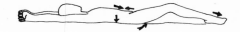

11. Hold Position #2. Raise one knee to your chest — hold. Then raise the other knee to your chest — hold.

12. **Stand, walk, and lift using this position always!**

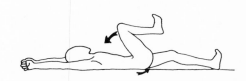

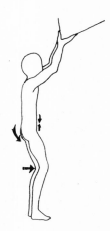

Alternate using Position #2 with the learning and practicing of the stretches, described in the next chapter, before you begin Position #3.

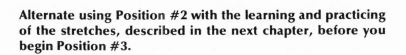

FIVE

The Stretches

If your back is hurting;
If you've been sitting too long;
If you've been in a car too long;
If you've been leaning over a sink;
If you got into the wrong position while sleeping;
If you've been wearing heels — no matter how you have misused yourself — it is time for one of the stretches. If one doesn't work, try another!

Be sure to inhale — and, as you exhale, let your back relax. You cannot relax completely without adding the breathing relaxation techniques.

As compression on your spine tries to force fluids out, extension of your spine tries to pull fluids in.

IMPORTANT   One of these stretches should become a part of your daily routine! Choose the sink or the overhead bar stretch.

Get into and out of the position several times every time you do it. Do this at least once or twice each day to create an alternating push-pull effect. This should help to maintain the elasticity of your spine and relieve the pressure on the discs. Repeat the stretch you choose. Stretch-relax-stretch-relax-stretch-relax each time you do it each day.

82

SINK STRETCHES

It is not unusual for people with low back pain to have a lot more pain when they lift their arms overhead, as in the overhead bar stretch. If you experience such an increase in pain, try this easier version of the stretch.

Locate a sturdy sink or something substantial attached to the wall. You might even try attaching a permanent bar to the wall, if you have the free wall space. Place your hands firmly around the bar at arms' length. Be sure your feet are directly under your shoulders.

Now bend your knees, tuck your bottom and your head under, let your hips lean slightly backward, and with small, careful side-to-side movements stretch your bottom toward the opposite wall. The farther you can ease your bottom backward and slightly downward, the more you are exerting traction — getting space between vertebrae where pressure is causing pain. Be sure to keep your lower back rounded as you stretch. Tuck your pelvis under more — bend your knees a little more — until the stretch feels just right for you.

Do at least three stretches at a time.

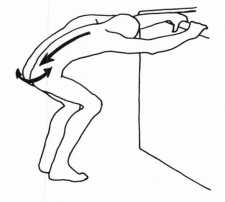

You will find that it will be easier for you to relax your lower back and to control it each time you repeat this exercise. You must relax your back *slowly* and repeatedly in order to permit extension of the discs.

Inhale, and then, as you exhale, let your back relax just a little. Keep repeating while in this position until you can release all the tension in your lower back. Use your hands to ease you back to standing. Then repeat the whole process. Then once again at least. This repetition allows your back to relax a little more each time.

Remember, releasing tension too fast can cause pain!

Release tension *slowly,* as in the other exercises. When the sink stretch feels comfortable, do the hip-movement exercises that follow. Doing them in conjunction with the sink stretches will increase movement in the lower spine and hip joints.

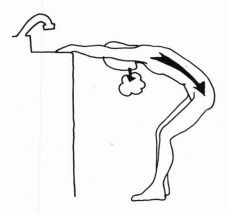

Do these stretches as soon as your back begins to hurt or feel tight. Make sure the sink you choose to use is firmly attached to the wall. Repeat the stretch you choose to do at least three times.

HIP FLEXIBILITY

Sometimes low back stiffness can be relieved by leaning on your forearms on a bureau, table, or some other stable piece of furniture, and keeping your feet on the floor while you walk in place.

Bend your knees and let your hips move up and down. It is the hip joints, knee joints, and lower back that need to be made mobile.

Do not let your whole body sway from side to side; such swaying will keep the movement in the lower back instead of allowing the hip joints to become loosened. Let the parts move very little to begin with; this will prevent nervousness and tension from making you tighten up even more.

Always start the movement gently and move into freer, more accentuated movements *slowly and cautiously*. The first few days you should be especially cautious. Use very gentle up-and-down movements.

It is going to take a little while for these areas (misuse of which can lead you into spasm) to adapt to the moves that will lead you to greater freedom in low back movement. Practically all people with low back pain learn to hold their lower backs in such a way as to avoid as much movement as they can, and learn to walk with as little hip movement as possible. This decreases general flexibility through all of these areas, makes you look and feel old, and doesn't improve anything.

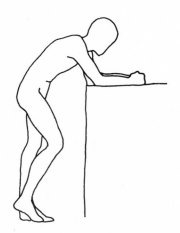

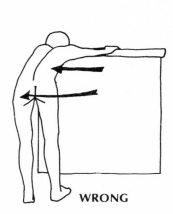

WRONG

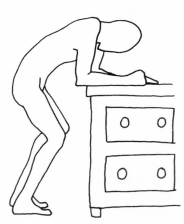

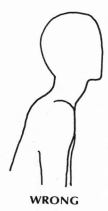 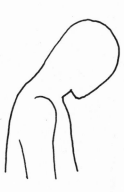

WRONG

It is important to choose a piece of furniture that is of the correct height to give you the most freedom from pain. A table may be the perfect height for one person to lean on, yet may cause pain to another. A bureau may suit the second person and bother the first.

Do not lean on your hands alone; lean on your forearms and hands. This, in most cases, will cause less pain. Your back as a whole tends to relax more when you place your arms on the surface you have chosen to lean on. Your back cannot relax if your head and neck are arched. Let your head and neck relax forward.

Make a conscious effort to relax all parts that you want to get moving. Trying to hold yourself so that you won't hurt is actually one of the ways in which, without meaning to, you cause yourself to go into even worse spasms!

IMPORTANT   Let go — relax — but gradually! In fact, you will find that you can probably let go completely, but if you do so too suddenly, you may cause yourself sharp and instant pain.

It is a mistake to cause yourself pain, but a mistake from which you can learn. You have to learn to be sneaky; let your back relax just a tiny bit at a time, until finally it is completely relaxed without your having caused yourself any pain at all!

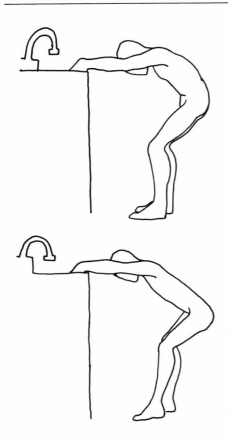

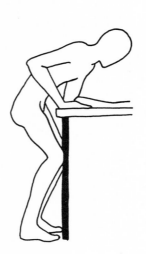

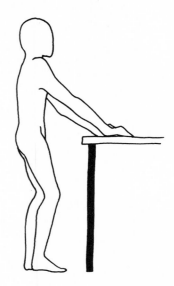

Time and practice should allow you to use all the parts of the intermittent rolling stretch which is the sink stretch combined with the hip movements and the roll from humped back to straight. It is an excellent three-way stretch for daily use.

ROLLING STRETCHES

As you progress with this exercise, you will find it helpful, after you have assumed the sink stretch position, to move your back gradually from a slightly humped position into a straight position, moving carefully and smoothly from one position to the other and back again, while continuing to let your hips go up and down.

When you are ready to stand straight after completing the exercise, raise your arms, leaving your hands on the surface of the table or bureau, and walk your hands — one after the other — to the edge of the surface closest to your body. This will put you in an upright position.

IMPORTANT Repeat the whole process at least three times. More is better. Don't let it hurt!

Stretch and relax — the combination of the stretching and relaxing is important — then the repetition of the combination of stretching and relaxing increases the good effect.

SITTING STRETCHES

If you have an overwhelming urge to stretch, try this. Sit on a chair or on the edge of your bed and stretch your arms and legs as far out in front of you as you can. Try to use all forward stretches as your *only* stretches until your back has been free of pain and discomfort for several months.

Think *"four-legged animal"*; our bodies (by the looks of them) are built to be safest in action when dealt with as if we *should* be on all fours. We are only slowly evolving to two-leggedness. That seems to be the reason that 80 percent of us have, at some time in our lives, problems with our lower backs.

It is up to you to protect your back! Most of your moves should be made in a forward direction.

Arching backward shortens the back muscles and puts the vertebrae in a less than protected position.

Stretch forward! Several times!

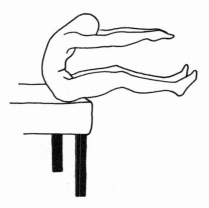

OVERHEAD BAR STRETCHES

If you get spasms in your back from sudden movement or from overdoing, you can often relieve the pain immediately. Remember that the sooner you perform this movement after the spasm begins, the more likely you are to relieve that spasm completely, immediately!

It is a mistake to let your back remain in spasm for even 5 minutes. The longer it is left unrelieved, the more muscles will become involved in the spasm, the more the injured tissues swell, and the longer it will take to get comfortable again.

IMPORTANT   The bar stretches, if done immediately, do the fastest and most complete job of relieving your sudden spasms!

First lie down in Position #1 so that when you stand you will be flexible enough to tuck and hold your pelvis under, keeping your knees just slightly bent.
Note: If your hands or arms are weak or if you are very overweight, this particular version may be impossible for you to do without experiencing more pain. See page 83.

If you have once had a spasm, you are likely to have others. Most people can tell when they are about to occur.

IMPORTANT   Whenever you anticipate a spasm, it is a useful idea to repeat this exercise. In any case, this is a good exercise for keeping your back relaxed and fighting the effect produced by gravity over the hours and over the years.

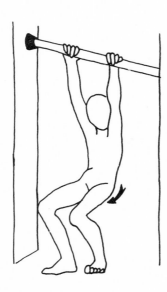

A "door-bar gym" which may be purchased in most sporting goods stores at a reasonable price, *or* just an ordinary piece of pipe put up with strong metal brackets in a door frame, is necessary for this exercise.

To judge the correct height of the door-bar gym, the person with a back problem should stand with knees bent, pelvis tucked under, and arms overhead. Remember that the bar or pipe should then be at the level where the person can grasp it comfortably while keeping the pelvis tucked under, knees bent, and feet *flat on the floor.*

IMPORTANT   Once the bar is in position (if it is the kind that clamps to the doorway), make sure someone else tests and tightens it every day.

If putting your arms overhead causes *more* pain, use the sink stretch only, or at least first.

Grasp the bar with your hands, and, making sure there is a pillow on the floor in front of your knees (for safety's sake), bend your knees and tuck your pelvis under. Keep the soles of your feet flat on the floor as you slowly and gently let all your weight hang from your hands.

If you feel your hands weakening *even a little* in their grasp, stand up immediately! **Take no chances of falling!**

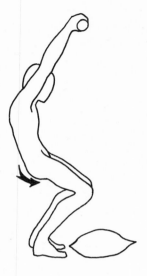

Hang in this position so that the weight of your hips, still tucked under, provides a *gentle* easing apart of the vertebrae, relieving the discs of compression.

If your hands or arms are beginning to feel the strain, *stand up slowly*. When you feel you can, get back into that position (it will take less time the second time around), and ease your hips down and under, from side to side, *very gently*. The hip action provides more pull, or traction, along the back than does simply hanging.

When your back feels eased or your arms feel too tired, stand; when you feel you can, repeat the exercise — and repeat — and repeat! Often you will actually feel the stretching and what *seems* to be something slipping back into place. If you do feel relief from pain, you have probably managed to ease your particular back problem for the moment.

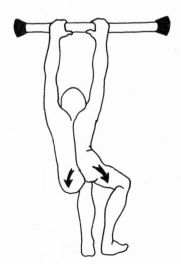

SIX

Position #3

Strange! On the one hand you may have heard that complete deep knee bends are harmful, and on the other hand you are told that you cannot pick up objects from the floor safely without squatting. The second statement is true!

IMPORTANT You cannot pick up objects from the floor safely without squatting!

Yet most men stop squatting as soon as they become involved daily in sedentary work, such as office work, driving cars or trucks, and other jobs that allow the thigh muscles to weaken.

Most women stop squatting as soon as they begin to wear girdles, or when the kids stop messing on the floor with one thing or another. Few people beyond the age of thirty-five squat even once a week! Even then, because of weakness of the thigh muscles, they tend to squat only while holding on to some stable object.

Not squatting weakens the whole pelvic area — not just the thighs. Your heel cords shorten, your knee ligaments become stiff, your balance in squatting is poor from lack of practice — and you are certainly going to have trouble lifting anything in so unstable a condition. You're going to need practice.

90

Position #3 is simply squatting with your pelvis tucked under, belly tight, feet lined up under knees.

Do not begin doing deep knee bends immediately! Unless you have been doing deep knee bends all along, the relearning, the increased flexibility, the strengthening, must be slow and gradual.

Being able to do deep knee bends gives you a much larger variety of movements, a much wider way of dealing with the world. Slowly deteriorating capabilities, unnoticeable in the beginning, suddenly shock and embarrass you when their absence is called to your attention.

IMPORTANT   If your thigh muscles are weak — if you seldom squat to do anything — you have become highly vulnerable to low back problems.

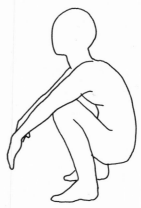

POSITION #3

DEEP KNEE BENDS

Even in cultures where squatting is a way of life — for defecating, for cooking, for tool-making, for the grinding of grains, for washing clothes — no one does 25 deep knee bends at a time!

It seems reasonable to suppose that once down and then up at a slower rate, with your lower back and your balance completely under control, will give you a good deal of work and will do so to better advantage.

PREPARING FOR POSITION #3

Obviously you are not going to be able to squat if you wear a girdle. Take it off!

Men and women both have trouble squatting if their slacks are too tight. Get into looser slacks or stretch ones.

Women won't want to squat in any case if they're wearing dresses. Get into slacks!

Balance is important in squats, as in everything else. Learn to squat *barefoot*, and hold on to something sturdy to keep your feet in line with your knees and to keep your feet apart to match the width of your hips.

If your knees tend to make cracking sounds when you squat or start to squat, it is wise to warm up your knees before you begin to bend them.

GAINING A "WELL-OILED" KNEE JOINT

IMPORTANT   If you haven't been doing many complete knee bends;

If your knees tend to crack when you bend even slightly;

If you have had knee problems at any time —

It is important to gain flexibility and increase circulation in your knee joint, well before you begin to add squats to your daily exercise!

Sit on the edge of a sturdy kitchen or dining room table. Let one lower leg swing like a pendulum from your knee.

IMPORTANT   If your knee feels at all uncomfortable, move your bottom either a little farther back or a little farther forward on the table and try the swinging again. You will find a point at which your lower leg will feel comfortable as it swings. Do the same with your other leg.

As you begin to feel more comfortable with your lower leg swinging, be sure — day by day — to move your bottom backward on the table. This gives you a wider arc through which your leg can swing.

This is an easy way to increase circulation and flexibility in your knee joint. Do it as much as you like.

It is a good idea to swing your leg in this manner a few times before you try your squats each day.

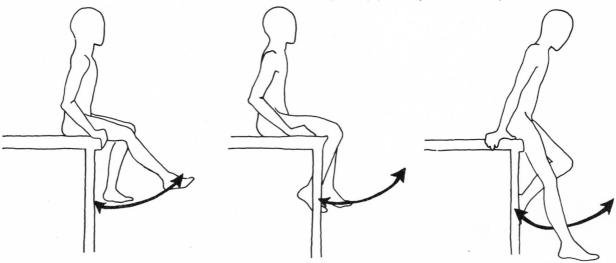

MAKING YOUR KNEES MORE FLEXIBLE

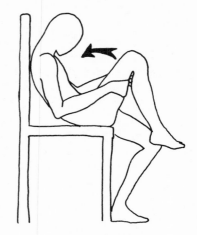

If when you are sitting you cannot fold each thigh up against your belly and chest and each lower leg against your thigh, you must first gain some flexibility before you will be able to squat.

After you "oil" your knee, sit in a chair in Position #1 — the modification for sitting (see page 129). Tighten your belly, put your hands *behind* one knee, and ease it closer, day by day, to your chest. Do the same with your other leg.

No forcing! Take your time!

Once your hip joint is flexible, it is time to go after your knee joint. Put your hands *around* one knee. Day by day, slowly ease your lower leg in against your thigh — closer and closer — until you can fold your thighs right in against your belly and chest and lower legs against your thighs. Once you can flex thigh to belly, leg to thigh, shift to using one hand around the knee, the other hand around the ball of your foot to start easing the whole of your foot in an upward direction toward your knee.

When your hips, knees, and feet seem completely flexible, with no weight on them, oil your knee again and start exercises, using your own body weight and thigh muscles in conjunction with the bending of your hips, knees, and ankles — *squatting!*

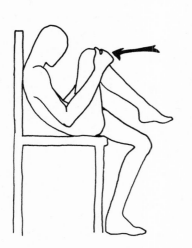

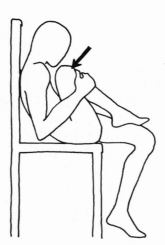

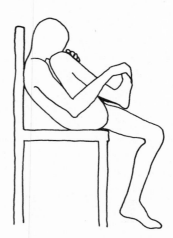

SITTING DOWN IN AND GETTING UP FROM A CHAIR

Start with two or even three cushions on the seat of a sturdy armchair that is facing a table.

Without using your hands, if possible, and without leaning forward, your feet hip-width apart, sit down in the chair, keeping one foot back under the chair and one foot forward, tighten your belly, tuck your bottom under, and get up again. Bring your knee directly forward over, or in line with, your foot. The table will give you something to grab hold of in case you have problems. Repeat this exercise several times the first day.

IMPORTANT   Try to raise and lower yourself more slowly every day.

Keep increasing the number of times until you can do 30 each day (spread them out over the day), using no hands.

IMPORTANT   Don't throw yourself forward! Momentum can hurt your back.

Take one cushion out and repeat the exercise. Start doing it a few times the first day, again working your way *slowly* up to 30 times daily. **Keep your bottom tucked under and tight!**

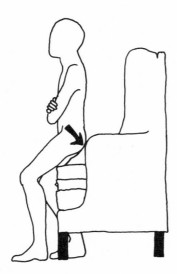

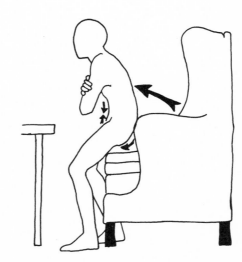

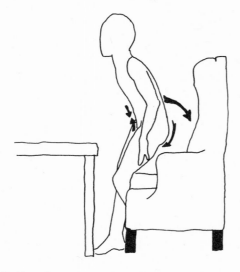 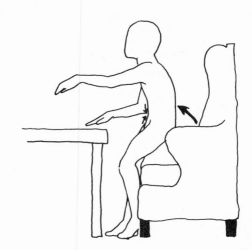

Take the last cushion out and begin again with a few repetitions of the exercise the first day. *Do them slowly!* Work your way up to 30 times daily again. **Keep your bottom tucked under and tight!**

IMPORTANT   Keep your feet apart to match the width of your hips. Your knees should move forward and back directly over your feet. Tighten your bottom and tuck it under! Keep your belly tight! Come up slowly and go down slowly.

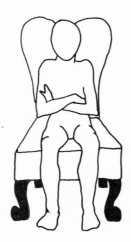

SQUATTING AND RISING

To get and keep your thighs very strong, try the following. Grab hold of the sink; then, with your knees and feet apart, tuck your bottom under, tighten your belly, and try a knee bend. *Go down slowly* — keeping your knees moving over your feet — no farther, at first, than just a little lower than a chair seat. *Come up slowly*, keeping your bottom tucked under.

IMPORTANT   Try to get a little farther down each day, but no more than you can manage in comfort. Don't force! Do it slowly.

Use the side of the sink for support as long as you need to. Then use the side of the sink only for balance, resting your fingertips on the edge. When you no longer need to rely on the sink, do your slow squatting with your feet apart, knees in line with your feet, using your arms out in front for balance and letting your heels come up off the floor. Rise up slowly. Sometimes just moving your feet a little farther apart will allow you to keep your heels down. Try, with time, to get your feet flat on the floor when you squat. (Rest your weight on the *outside* edges of your feet!)

Want to go further?

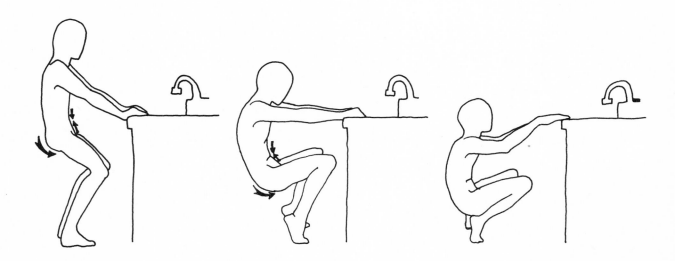

Try sitting down slowly into a squat and getting up slowly without using your hands, until finally you can come up 30 times in one day, always in the right position.

IMPORTANT   Keep your feet apart to match the width of your hips. Your knees move forward and back along lines that point in the same direction as your feet. Tighten your bottom and tuck it under! Keep your belly tight! Come up slowly and go down slowly!

Want to go further? Don't try it until you've been completely free of pain for at least a month!

Cross your feet and come down to the floor onto your bottom and then stand up. Can you make it? Thirty times in one day? *If you have trouble getting back up,* lean back just a little, your arms up, *belly tight,* and then *lean your arms and body forward for counterbalance, purse your mouth, breathe out,* and lift yourself up.

IMPORTANT   Don't use momentum! Use your belly and thigh strength. Rise forward and up — slowly and steadily. Don't let yourself fall!

Try using the floor more for your sitting. Get out of the habit of using your hands to get up.

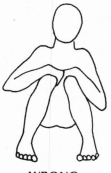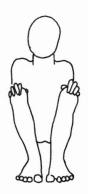

WRONG

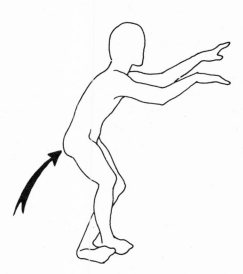

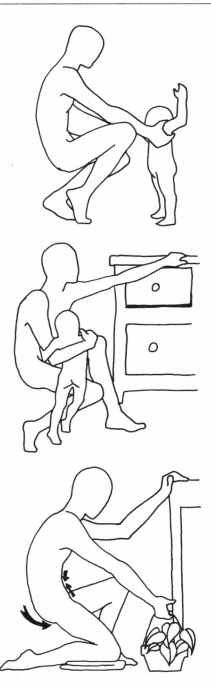

Variations on Squatting

To accommodate those who have knee, hip, or foot problems — those whose balance may not be up to par — here
are some variations you can use in squatting. Use those that
feel most comfortable for you.

**IMPORTANT   Keep your feet apart to match the width of
your hips. Your knees should move forward and back in a
line directly over your feet. Tighten your bottom and tuck it
under! Keep your belly tight! Come up slowly and go down
slowly!**

Let your heels come up off the floor if you feel unstable
with them flat.

Sometimes you may find that having one foot forward and
one foot back will make squatting much easier for you.

It may be that you can lift to better advantage if you have
one foot flat on the floor and the other foot with the heel
raised.

**IMPORTANT   It is important for your back and for your legs
that you learn to squat!**

**If you can never squat without holding on, then squat —
and hold on!**

You will often find it more comfortable to kneel with one
leg. (Always put a rug or a pillow or folded towel under your
knee.)

A heavy table or a wall on one side of you will give you the
needed support for one hand if the object you are picking
up turns out to be heavier than you expected.

**IMPORTANT   Always! Forevermore! Every single time you
start to lift while squatting or to rise from squatting, tighten
your belly and tuck your bottom under before you start up!**

Position #3 Check List

This check list is for after you have worked your way up to — and have gotten back to — comfortably squatting again:

1. Sit on the edge of a table — or just stand — and swing your lower leg 30 times from the knee.
2. Then standing — Tuck! Tighten! Clench!
3. — and slowly squat!
   — leaning very slightly forward,
   — preferably barefoot,
   — knees moving out over your feet.
4. Tuck! Tighten! Clench!
   — and leaning slightly forward,
   slowly rise!

Do this *at least* 5 or 6 times each day!

IMPORTANT   Keep your feet the width of your hips apart! Your knees move forward and back along lines that point in the same directions as your feet! Tighten your bottom and tuck it under! Keep your belly tight! Come up slowly and go down slowly!

It is important for your back and for your legs to squat! If you can never squat without holding on, then squat! — and hold on!

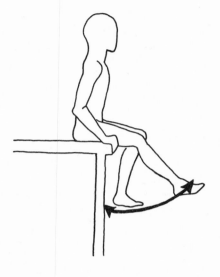

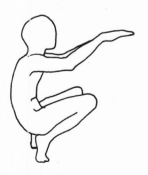

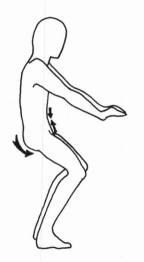

SEVEN

Exercises for Particular Pain

SCIATIC PAIN

So-called sciatica is what you feel when the sciatic nerve becomes irritated. The irritation can be caused by anything that exerts pressure on the sciatic nerve or on the nerve roots of the spinal cord that combine to form the nerve. When the nerve is irritated in any one place, it tends to become irritable everywhere else along its course.

Keep all hard or lumpy objects out of your hip pockets. Sitting on chairs with raised edges can irritate the nerve. Lumpy seats can irritate the nerve. Sitting on cold concrete can irritate the nerve. Overstretching or stretching too quickly can irritate the nerve. Low car seats can irritate the nerve. Bottom muscles so loose and underdeveloped that they flatten out can allow pressure to irritate the nerve. Too little fat to pad the bottom can allow the nerve to be irritated easily. Sitting too long on a toilet seat or straining to have a bowel movement can irritate the nerve. Cutting down the local circulation and applying pressure by crossing your legs can irritate the nerve by stretching it. Overweight and carrying things that are too heavy for you can put pressure on the nerve. **Low back problems can irritate the nerve!** All of the above can cause further irritation in a nerve already sensitive from low back problems.

1. If your bottom is flabby, begin to build it up by clenching it (Position #2).
2. If your bottom is bony because your are underweight, put on weight in the form of muscle by eating a good, high protein diet.
3. Sit on surfaces that are neither cold nor hard.
4. Stand (but keep moving!) rather than sitting still.
5. Keep your bowels regular.
6. Keep your legs uncrossed.
7. Take walks.
8. Start an exercise program slowly and work up gradually. The only remedy I have ever heard of that actually made sciatic pain disappear reasonably fast is mild exercise. The exercises for *low back problems*, combined with a gradually increased *walking program* using good posture, seem to work best.

A good walking program calls for you to walk until you reach just this side of pain. Then rest. Repeat at intervals during the day. Sometimes it takes weeks for the pain to disappear completely. But you will find that you can walk a little farther each day before the pain begins. *It is important that you walk properly if you are going to achieve the proper results* (see pages 75–79).

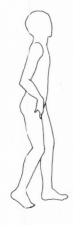

PAINFUL HIP JOINT

If one of your hip joints is aching because you constantly rest your weight on it, or even for unknown reasons, this is the exercise that will probably help the most.

Stand on a stool or sideways on the bottom step of your stairs, with your leg hanging free from the painful hip. Lean forward until you can rest your arms comfortably against a chair or the bannister. This helps prevent your arching your back when you let your leg swing to the rear. It will also place the end of your thigh bone in the freest position in the socket of the hip.

Try to get your hanging leg to feel as if it isn't yours; just let it hang there limply. Give it enough of a swing to get it started, and let it swing freely — only back and forth. *Do not swing your leg to the side, as this will pull at your back!* Get it hanging really heavily from your hip.

IMPORTANT   Do not use your leg muscles to help your leg swing! It must swing like a pendulum.

The weight of your hanging leg will cause some extension in the soft material of the hip joint, and will usually serve to relieve some or all of your pain.

Try not to repeat those positions that caused the pain.

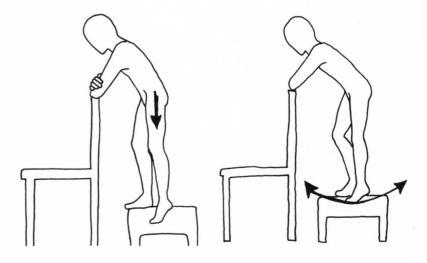

EIGHT

Conditions That Make Back Pain Worse

OVERWEIGHT

Carrying extra weight is absolutely foolhardy when your back is weak or painful! It takes little extra weight to put added compression on the discs of your lower back. Worse yet is the effect of the extra weight on your belly muscles, which are probably already weak.

If your belly sticks out even a little, gravity can drag it down. That gives you not only weakness to fight, but also gravity. Double trouble! Keep adding more weight, and the belly — muscles, fat, and all — begins to sag more and more, until it finally rolls over the top of your thighs and your problem gets worse and worse. For most people the farther the belly protrudes and sags, the more the lower back is going to hurt!

It is absolutely necessary that you begin working on your belly muscles immediately and that gradually and steadily you try to get your weight under control. In any case, what you do now is important. Several times every day stretch yourself out with Position #1. Don't let the pain begin in your lower back; if it's already there, don't let it get worse!

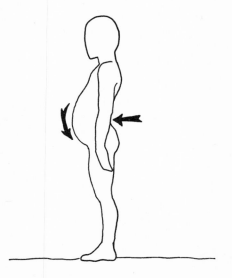

IRREGULARITY

The increased pressure in the lower belly from constipation, even from the daily accumulation in the bowels waiting to be expelled normally, can cause much increased low back pain. Many people find that their low back pain is much relieved immediately after defecation. Constipation presents a worse problem. The hardened matter produces more pressure against the lower back, enough to cause, sometimes, severe pain. The job of forcing it out can be enough to wreck your lower back for the day, if not longer. It becomes terribly important to keep your bowels open and the movement as push-free as possible if you are going to prevent further pain. This does not mean that you should take laxatives! Now is the time to learn how to adjust the roughage in your diet for achieving the right consistency of the waste matter.

How long have you been taking laxatives? A year? Longer? It makes no difference. There are very few people who can't beat the laxative habit. The reason you start taking laxatives is that you lack things that are essential to living: sufficient roughage, sufficient fats and oils, and sufficient physical activity.

In the colon (the final section of the intestines) there is carried on both extraction of water from the wastes and also what is called "peristaltic action" (the "milking" action that works the wastes along the intestines). When only refined foods are eaten, there is no bulk left when water is extracted and it becomes more and more difficult for the wastes to move along.

Salads and fresh fruits are good roughage; seeds and nuts are better; bran and the outer covering of rice and other grains are good, but sometimes *too* rough alone to be usable by those of you who have made your colons delicate with the use of refined foods. Rushing food that is already impaired by being too refined through your system with laxatives does not allow it time to be properly dehydrated by your colon. Unrefined foods tend to have more roughage; this increases digestion time and spreads out the digestive work in your stomach and intestines. Digestion takes time. Your health depends on your giving your body the food —

and the time — it takes to do the best job. Seeds and nuts are not only high in nutritional value, but also require chewing and supply roughage. Lack of teeth almost invariably leads to one's eating only refined foods. Eating refined foods almost invariably leads to lack of teeth. Chewing supplies the pressure teeth and jawbones need to remain healthy.

SEED CEREAL

Mix together: 1 lb. sunflower seed meal or whole seeds
1 lb. pumpkin seed meal or whole seeds
1 lb. sesame seeds, unhulled
1 lb. wheat germ, toasted or untoasted
1 lb. noninstant powdered milk
1 lb. date chips, raisins, date sugar, or chopped apricots
1 lb. broken pecans or other nuts

— and keep refrigerated in tightly covered canister.

1. Use with milk or yogurt as cereal.

2. Date chips or another fruit serve as sweetener. Use or leave out, as you like.

3. One cup of mixture with 1 teaspoon of baking powder and a pinch of salt mixed in, to which is added 1 egg and enough milk to bring to batter consistency, can be baked on a cast-iron or other type pan to make great pancakes.

Variation: Leave out baking powder and fold in 2 stiffly beaten egg whites.

Variation: If you can't chew comfortably, put seeds and fruits through blender; then let soak 5 to 15 minutes in fruit juice, milk, or yogurt.

A quarter of a cup of this seed cereal, with milk added immediately before serving, if chewed very well, should in time solve most constipation problems.

If you take laxatives every day, continue to take them every day the first week that you eat this cereal daily. The second week, continue to eat the cereal every day, but take the laxatives only every other day.

On the days you don't take the laxative, do the following. Before getting *out* of bed, bend your knees, place your feet on the bed and arms at your sides, put a pillow or pillows under your head and shoulders, a pillow or pillows under your knees and hips — then loosely "blop" your belly in and out about 20 to 50 times. Pull in and push up with your innards. This helps to get the peristaltic action going.

Then drink one full glass of hot water (with a little lemon juice if you want), and complete your usual morning routine and breakfast. Don't worry if you don't have a bowel movement on these in-between days. Remember, it takes around 24 hours for you to put enough into the colon to *have* a bowel movement!

The third week, try two consecutive days off the laxatives — doing belly bloppers — and one day on laxatives. Take the seed cereal every day. If you get lazy about the seed cereal at this stage, you may upset the whole system and have to start over. Keep right with it! It's a marvelous feeling to have your body doing its own work again — and certainly much more healthful for you and your back!

The fourth week, take the laxative only two days and do so only if the adjustment of your system to the new way of doing things is slow. If you do feel that the changeover is slow, do belly-blopping in the right position night *and* morning for a few weeks. It's worth the extra effort!

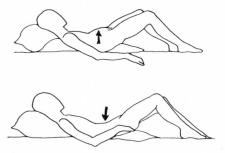

ONE SHORT LEG

Only your doctor can tell you if you have one leg that is shorter than the other. The measurement has to be taken from an x-ray while you are standing with hips even, feet a few inches apart. A spasm, scoliosis (a structural defect of the spine), or other problems can give you the *appearance* of a short leg, without your really having one. On the other hand, one cause of scoliosis *is* the unequal length of the legs. A wrong step in trying for correction can give you even more problems. Be sure to consult your doctor!

I have personally seen a maximum of three quarters of an inch added to the useful and apparent length of a short leg by means of the following exercise!

Stand on the bottom step of your stairs (a box near a bureau will do). Lean slightly *forward* to prevent your lower back from arching as you swing your leg back. Lean with your hands or arms on the bannister or bureau. Your shorter leg is left hanging free.

Start with an easy pendulumlike movement, letting your leg hang heavily from your hip joint.

After a few days, when you feel you have an easy swing, with your leg *not* pulling *up* into your hip joint, add a *small* weight to your ankle. Some tools tied into a handkerchief or rag are good enough. A half-pound weight is not too small! There must be very gradual increases of the weight over a period of weeks.

To save yourself problems, do not increase the weight more often than once a week! Do not increase the weights too rapidly! The tissue can be overstretched if the weight is made too heavy, too fast. Or your hip muscles may react automatically to pull your hip back into the joint, thereby preventing the easy stretching that you need.

IMPORTANT   Let your leg hang limp! Use your leg like a pendulum. Do not try to hurry this exercise! Do not try to be energetic as you perform this movement!

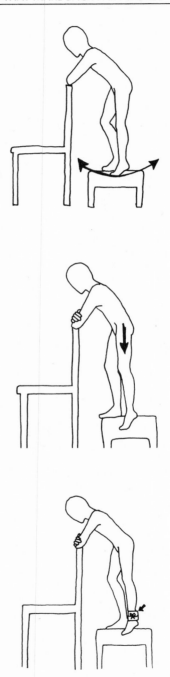

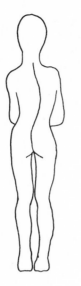

SCOLIOSIS

Scoliosis can cause low back pain, or can be caused by low back pain. In a simple scoliosis, the spine makes an s-curve. Usually it bends to the right side (as we look at the back from behind) just under the shoulder blades, then curves over a little too far to the left at the lower back.

You can be born with this problem. You can develop it after birth. It can be caused by missing muscles (not all of us have the full complement of muscles). It can develop because of a short leg. It can develop by your trying to protect yourself from low back pain. It can be caused by deformed or deforming vertebrae. It can be caused by severe muscle spasms. It can be caused by poor habits of posture. It can be caused by uneven muscular strength.

Posture and gravity have an enormous influence on your spine. A spine that is already sinking to the side will sink more under the pressure of gravity. Unless you have, or are willing to develop, the right habits to fight further changes, a mild scoliosis can become a severe scoliosis in ten years! A severe scoliosis can take form in a few years during the early teens, when growth is rapid.

One of the simplest methods for effecting change can be used while you sleep!

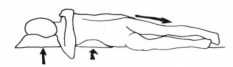

Lie on the side that bulges most under your arm. Have one pillow under your head and another small pillow or folded towel under the bulge itself. This will line up your spine better through the rib cage area. Then stretch your hip out along the bed to straighten the spine through the pelvis as much as possible. You can combine this with Position #1.

Nightly reminders to yourself to roll back into position when you roll off the pillow will soon get you into the *habit* of sleeping in a position that will allow your spine to relax into a more correct alignment.

If you have had scoliosis for many years and have not done anything to combat it, you must begin at whatever level you can and work your way as far as you can! Real determination can, at the very least, prevent the curves from getting worse. Once your back is no longer painful, you can try swimming; it will allow you to use your muscles evenly while your spine is supported by the water. If you can arrange to swim every day (really swim — do not float or rest)

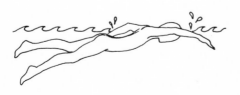

for an hour, you may be able to prevent the scoliosis from getting worse. Of course, swimming will keep your whole body in very good condition. Take a friend and make it your daily treat!

If you are a young or active person with scoliosis but no low back pain, you will find that overhead rings, the trapeze, parallel bar, or ladder will allow you to align and strengthen your whole body and to extend your spine. Extension helps the spine to unwind its twistings — like letting the receiver of your telephone hang free to unwind the cord. The bars and trapezes are not the kind of equipment that is easily available for use once you are out of school unless you have it installed at home. If you have scoliosis, it's worth installing. A ladder attached overhead down a hall would do. If you cannot afford to have the equipment installed, look for a gym that has the equipment — and a trainer, as well.

To ease scoliosis strain during the day, rest your hand against your rib cage right where it bulges out, and either push *gently* in against the bulge, or lean your elbow into the chair or sofa that you're sitting in or the wall that you are close to — until you feel your spine being eased back toward the right position. This is especially good to do right after you do the sink or overhead bar stretch.

But don't wait! Do it as often as you think of it or as often as you can!

You may want to put counterpressure on the opposite side of the bulge, with your hand on your neck to prevent your head from remaining out of line with the rest of your body.

Don't do it if it makes you dizzy!

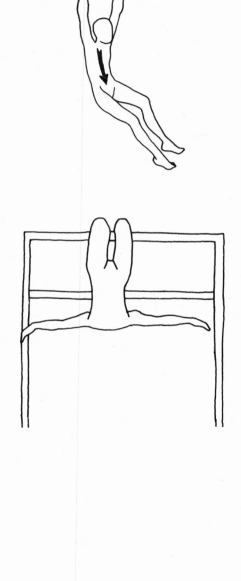

NINE

Women's Matters

There are some problems that only women have. This chapter is especially designed for those women who have low back pain.

IMPORTANT   But first: have you had a gynecological check-up? A large percentage of backaches in women are caused by gynecological complaints. Don't take it for granted that there is another cause. Check it out!

MENSTRUATION

Just before menstruation, the uterus, as its walls become heavier, sometimes puts pressure on your lower back. It also sets up what is called "referred" pain. *Menstrual periods almost invariably will make a low back problem worse!*

Most women retain extra fluids throughout the body at this time. The belly almost always feels bloated. *There is usually a weight gain of anywhere from 3 to 10 pounds at this time!*

A help can be the high protein diet given later in this chapter. It will keep you from carrying a lot of those extra fluids!

**IMPORTANT   During menstruation, pregnancy, and meno-
pause, the tone of the colon and the tone of the belly muscles get weaker. Your belly is hanging out!**

This produces a further stress on your lower back. It is important to develop very strong belly muscles — strong to
the point that, in spite of the lowering of tone, you can still
exert control over how far out your belly goes.

**IMPORTANT   Be aware that the loss of tone in your colon
means you may have further problems with constipation or
simply with slowed-down evacuation. Keep the roughage in
your diet high! (See pages 104–105).**

TEN-DAY MENSTRUAL DIET

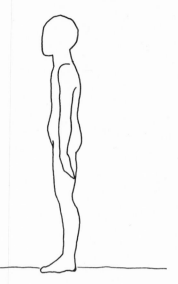

You should start this diet five days before your period
begins and continue it for the next five days. The liver, parsley, and sardines will help keep your iron level up. (Most
menstruating women are anemic until menopause, and con-
sequently feel tired and weak.) This diet should help give
you better control of your belly muscles and, therefore, of
your back, because the roughage will encourage good movement of the bowels and the high protein level will lessen
fluid retention. The high calcium level will probably help
you to feel more cheerful and calm, and is conducive to a
lessening of pain.

All the nutritional information in this diet comes from two
government books, which can be ordered from the accom-
panying addresses. Inquire about charges and send for:

1 *Composition of Foods — Agricultural Handbook No. 8*
   Superintendent of Documents
   U.S. Government Printing Office
   Washington, D.C. 20402
2 *Recommended Dietary Allowances*
   National Academy of Sciences
   2101 Constitution Avenue
   Washington, D.C. 20418

Breakfast:
Protein, 10 grams; calories, 228.
1 cup hot water with the juice of 1/4 lemon
1 oz. (or 1/8 cup or 3 heaping tbsp.) toasted or plain wheat

germ (add 1 tbsp. bran as you need to for better bowel movements)
8 oz. skim milk, for cereal and/or drinking
1/2 banana
cups of hot or cold lemon water, as needed

Lunch:
Protein, 20 grams; calories, 175.
cups of hot or cold water, as needed
4 oz. (or 1/2 cup) packed cottage cheese or 1 small can sardines
10 leaves or 1/4 head loose-leaf lettuce
1 tbsp. oil
2 or 3 sprigs of parsley
cups of hot or cold water, as needed

Dinner:
Protein, 25 grams; calories, 225.
cups of hot or cold water, as needed
1/4 pound liver, any kind
1 tbsp. butter
1 green pepper
10 leaves or 1/4 head loose-leaf lettuce
cups of hot or cold lemon water, as needed

Snack:
Protein, 7 grams; calories, 72.
8 oz. skim milk

**Total protein, about 71 grams;
total calories, about 710.**

For best results — no additions, no subtractions, and no substitutions!

TAMPONS

Most women can use tampons with no trouble, but some women cannot use tampons of any kind because they cause back pain.

Quite a few women think that their back pain is due to their menstrual period and never realize that a simple shift to sanitary napkins might solve the problem for them.

Exercising when you are wearing a tampon can again be a

cause of low back pain. Don't blame the pain on your body until you have checked every other possibility.

Look also to diaphragms and IUDs as *possible* causes of your low back pain. Each individual's sensitivity level is different!

PREGNANT?

During pregnancy, you experience several changes that can give you problems with your back. All these changes can be dealt with.

1. Your uterus and the fetus begin to increase in size and weight, and pull on the ligaments by which the uterus is supported from the back.
2. Your body retains more fluids.
3. The tone of your belly muscles and colon lessens, making it difficult to hold your belly in and easy to become constipated.
4. Changing balance as your belly enlarges causes you to lean back from your hips if your belly and bottom muscles are not kept very strong.
5. Your balance changes from moment to moment as the baby moves. Keep moving! Constant movement accustoms you to dealing with the changing balance.

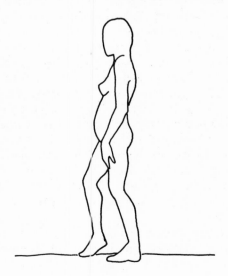

POSTNATAL BACK

Just had a baby? During the last period of pregnancy, hormonal activity causes the ligaments of your pelvis to become more elastic. It also loosens ligaments elsewhere in your body. This allows your pelvis to stretch to some extent when the baby is forced through. The baby gives a little; your pelvis gives a little.

If you are healthy and move well in ways that will strengthen the muscles of your pelvis and belly, these ligaments will usually tighten up once more to give you a strong pelvis and lower back after your baby is born. If the ligaments stay loose, just a very small weakness may cause problems to develop either soon after delivery or even some years later. Quite often, weaknesses that occur during pregnancy are not recognized as the causes of later problems.

The worst postpregnancy problem is traditional but can be changed rapidly. The height and the form of cribs could have been designed by a hater of mothers! The angle at which you have to lean, the impossibility of bending a leg to tilt the pelvis to arrange yourself for lifting, puts your back in the position most conducive to encouraging low back weakness and pain.

The hospital crib, on the other hand, is well designed. It is high enough so you do not have to lean over to tend the baby, though it would be better still if it had a strong rung underneath on which you could put one foot.

Prevention of the above problems is simple. Take a long bureau drawer and put it on top of a low bureau or a table that you have covered with a nonskid foam pad. Use the drawer instead of a crib! Your arms should be able to lift the baby, change his or her diapers, change the bedding, without your having to bend forward from the hips at all!

To safeguard further your low back area, put a box about eight to twelve inches high by the side of the bureau or under the table, and put one foot up on it when you have to work by the makeshift bed. This helps tilt your pelvis just enough to put it in a position that will prevent any strain on your lower back.

If, in spite of knowing its faults, you are still going to use a crib, raise the mattress as high as possible, making sure you

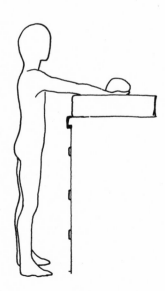

WRONG

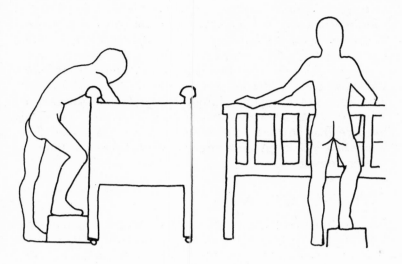

leave a good distance between the top of the mattress and the railing, and put a box, on which to rest one foot, in front of the crib.

You will learn by experience whether you relieve your back more by placing the left or the right foot on the box. Maybe changing feet from time to time will help even more. Use the hand on the side opposite the foot you are going to raise to stabilize you as you *tighten your bottom and belly* to lift your leg up! Rubber stoppers or a rubber mat will prevent the box's slipping from under your foot.

Now is the time — right after you've had your baby — to retighten your belly muscles, pulling your pelvis firmly up in front with elastic belly muscles and a flexible back. You will achieve this most easily if you worked during your pregnancy to keep your lower belly wall as tight and as strong as you could, and your back flexible, with your pelvis tucked under. This will make recovery after pregnancy totally simple, as it will be a continuation of habits already developed!

Care and thought have to be given to how and when you begin to exercise after delivery. Your doctor, if you had one, may be your guide. If you are going to proceed on your own, you *must* do so with the greatest caution. If you had a caesarean section, if you hemorrhaged, move *extremely cautiously* into only the simplest movements, such as lying with your knees bent and breathing out with your mouth pursed.

Do not take chances! **Moving too quickly into strong exercises may cause setbacks.** A wait of two weeks or longer, if advised, is not going to do long-term damage. In any case, it is better to take a few steps back into far easier exercises and be sure that you are safe, than to try the hard exercises immediately or even soon after delivery. Take your time — just be consistent!

PUTTING ON A BRA

Put the bra that fastens in the back around you back-to-front; fasten the closings while they are in front of you; then slide the bra around to the back and slip the straps up over your shoulders!

Or, first put the straps over your shoulders. Put one hand onto a bureau or the headboard of your bed to steady yourself if you need to. Put one foot up on the bed; then lean forward to let your breasts fill the cups of the brassiere. Fasten it *while you remain in this position*. Straighten your back and take your foot down!

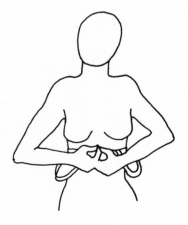
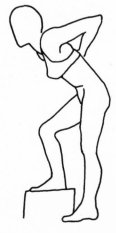

WEARING SLACKS FOR SQUATTING AND LIFTING

("I see London, I see France . . .")

A female's pelvis is wider than a male's; this means that for balance and safety a female's feet should be slightly farther apart, in line with her hips, when she is squatting. The knees should be in line with the feet, to prevent knee problems. An object to be lifted must be pulled in *close to the body* — between the legs!

Even very young girls are taught to keep their knees together, especially when squatting. This wrecks balance, places stress on knees, and puts a twist in the disc material as it forces a dangerous one-sided lift.

Habits are harder to change as we practice them. How much better to allow young girls the same chance as boys to have healthy backs! A simple change from dresses to slacks makes it easy!

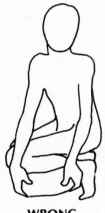 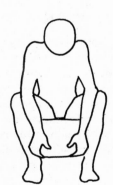

WRONG

TEN

Coping with Everyday Life

KEEPING WARM

Your body temperature can be lowered by
cold water,   cold weather,
a breeze,   lying still,
a cold house,   sleeping.

Every muscle is made up of a lot of muscle fibers. The power a muscle exerts depends on how many fibers are contracting (actually, they twitch) at the same time.

When the muscle is pulling hard, as it is when you lift, many of the fibers are contracting at the same time. *But even when the muscle is resting, some of the fibers are contracting.* When more of the fibers are contracting at rest, there is an *increase* in resting tone. Your muscles increase their tone in order to produce heat to try to keep your body warm. This makes you feel stiff — or may even make you shiver — and can cause more pain in your lower back.

When fewer of the fibers are contracting at rest, there is a *decrease* in resting tone. Heat from outside the body relieves the muscles of the work of keeping you warm and allows them to relax.

Try:

a warmer house,   a warm bath,
warmer clothing,   or a heating pad,
warmer bedclothes,   or a hot water bottle.

Taking a Bath

One good way to relieve low back pain is to take a warm
bath. Try to get someone to run the water and help you ease
yourself into the tub. Bring warm clothes into the bathroom
so that you can change into them before leaving the warm
air. Make sure the temperature of the water feels quite
warm, but *not hot*. Keep the bathroom door closed so that
room temperature will be raised and there will be no cold air
to cause spasms when you leave the tub. Place towels over
the radiator before you get into the tub so that they will be
warm when you dry yourself, or put them in a slightly warm
oven and arrange for someone to bring them to you when
you are ready.

Once you are sitting in the tub, ease yourself down until
your lower back is rounded. If your back is hurting badly,
stay in that position for a few minutes to give the spasm time
to ease a little. You can *help ease the spasm by inhaling and,
as you exhale, consciously relaxing your back*. Be sure to
keep the temperature in the tub warm by adding, or having
some else add, hot water from time to time.

As your back relaxes, you may get a sudden increase of
pain; it could be only that you have relaxed your back too
fast. Repeat the inhaling and exhaling for relaxing but control the relaxing, letting your back ease slowly and gently. If
you don't seem to be able to relax your back this way, it may

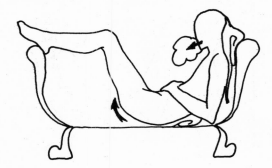

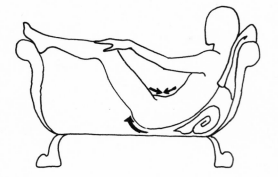 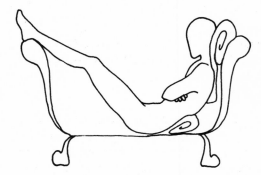

mean that you are in the wrong position. Brace the soles of your feet against the end of the tub, with your arms on the sides of the tub. Tighten your belly muscles and lift your bottom slightly, enough to tighten it and rotate it under, and rest the bony area of your back (the sacrum) on the bottom of the tub. A folded towel in the tub behind your lower back will support it and should help ease your pain.

A folded towel under your head will help you keep your chin close to your chest. According to the length of your body and the right position for you, your feet may be placed up against the end of the tub, over the edge of the tub, or even up on the wall behind the end of the tub. Putting your feet over the edge of the tub is least likely to be helpful;

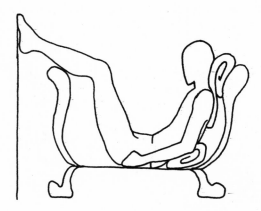

supporting the soles of your feet on the tub helps you hold your position so that you are not likely to slip under the water.

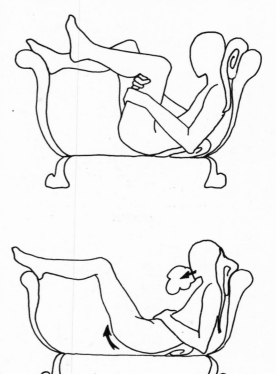

As in all other positions of comfort for low back problems, you must keep your back rounded, with your chin and knees only as close to your chest as is comfortable. **Do not just lie there.** *Ease* one knee up toward your chest *gently* by using both hands slipped behind the knee. Ease up one knee at a time, supporting yourself with the other foot against the end of the tub. **Don't try to stretch too far!** Then keep your hands under your knee as you ease your foot back toward the end of the tub. Do the same thing for the other leg.

While in the tub, you may try Position #2. Very slowly and gently tighten just your bottom muscles, exhaling through your pursed mouth at the same time. Hold as long as possible and then relax those muscles as slowly as possible. When you're ready to leave the tub, call for someone to help you out and to empty and clean the tub for you. Doing this yourself can often undo all the good work you did for your back in the tub!

IMPORTANT   If you need a lot of help to get into and out of the tub, if using the tub makes your back more painful, stick with using heat in bed while in Position #1.

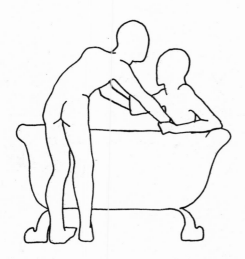

Sleeping Warm

When you sleep, your body temperature drops. When your body temperature drops, your connective tissue becomes less elastic. Muscles increase their tone to try to keep you warm. If your back is in a position that causes the discs to be compressed, the tightening can cause you yet more discomfort or pain. Position #1 is basic!

Warm clothes will help. Keep your back, especially the length of your spine, completely covered. A slight stiffening anywhere on your spine can cause a reaction along the rest of it.

An electric blanket is sheer luxury! It may be a terrible waste of energy, but it is a positive release from pain for many people! Preventing the drop in body temperature can, for some people, make the difference between sleep and restlessness. If you have pain while sleeping that is not relieved with reasonable ease by Position #1 alone, try an electric blanket.

If you can't afford or don't like an electric blanket, wear your old woolen sweaters, old sweat suits, jersey slacks — in layers. Especially if you have low back pain, a blanket that doesn't tuck closely in around *you* (not the mattress) just doesn't do the trick. Make sure the sweaters are long enough to prevent a gap at the back of your waist when you are in Position #1! (Women — try dresses of wool knit over your slacks.)

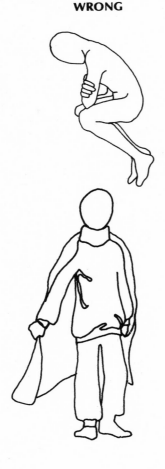

WRONG

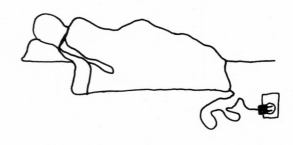

Using a Heating Pad or a Hot Water Bottle

Heat is to be used only after diagnosis of your low back pain and with your doctor's okay! Heat acts to increase local circulation *and as a counterirritant*. Because it is hard for a person to notice two sensations at the same time, the feeling of heat counteracts the feeling of pain.

Try it for yourself. If you pinch your arm hard enough to make it hurt more than your back hurts, you cannot at the same time notice the pain in your back. Some doctors use this method when giving injections. Women in delivery are taught to give so much of their attention to a particular way of breathing that they can handle the discomfort of childbirth.

IMPORTANT The problem involved when using heat is that, if your back pain is bad enough, you may use a heating pad that is so hot that it can burn your skin before you stop noticing the pain in your back.

It is safer — much safer — to use a hot water bottle containing water no hotter than your hand can stand to remain in for any length of time. *Always wrap the hot water bottle in a towel!* A combination of the heat and Position #1, used always with the breathing for relaxing, should relieve your pain without causing injury.

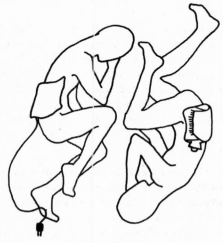

WRONG

BEDS

How many hours a day do you spend in bed? One third of your life is the average. **That's a lot of time!**

You may be asleep, but you are still alive. Make your bed as luxurious as you can — not in looks, though that's all right — but in *comfort!*

You spend hours — days — looking for a car you spend only a small part of your day in, and usually spend a small fortune on! A bed is generally kept a lot longer than a car. It should be the most comfortable one you can afford.

Enjoying your bed helps you to sleep and rest better. It improves the quality of your whole day — your whole life! Treat yourself well. You deserve it!

If you have a painful lower back, a hard bed is not necessarily right for you. We differ in our reactions to different surfaces — and we differ greatly in body shape and weight.

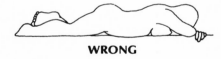

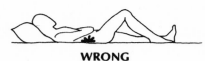

WRONG

A man with a large belly may find that lying on his belly actually brings relief from back pain, because the areas in which the fat is distributed curve his back out rather than letting it sag into an arch. Someone with a flat belly, lying in the same position, would have pain because the back would arch. A woman with a large belly and still larger breasts may find that, if she lies on her belly, her breasts may let her lower back sag, causing pain. Most people who are overweight, in fact, are very uncomfortable sleeping on their bellies. As you can see, it is not the surface that is important; it is a matter of whether the spine can be held straight in a curled or fetal position. I tend to favor a bed with a soft surface rather than a hard one for a specific reason. If the person with the lower back problem can lie comfortably only on his back, any tender surface spots on the back are going to be forced into the surface of the bed to some extent. Do you want a painful area forced into a hard surface or into a giving surface?

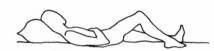

WRONG

IMPORTANT   If your back is in pain, it is very difficult to come into contact with a surface that does not give. It is not ever necessary to lie on a hard surface unless it positively eases the pain for you! A hard surface does not ease most people's pain! Those points on their backs that are tender are pressed into the hard surface, causing more pain.

A *sagging mattress* is bad for your back. But this does not mean that you must necessarily go to the opposite extreme — a hard mattress — to try to be comfortable! Many people find that a bed that does not sag and has a soft flat surface gives them greater freedom from pain than one with a hard flat surface.

Only because a hard bed is better than a *sagging* bed, people assume that it is better for them than a soft one. It is difficult to try out different surfaces until you find what *is* comfortable for you.

If you have a mattress that sags because of the bed frame or springs, try putting a three-quarter-inch board under the mattress to support it on an even level. This may be the only change you need. If you are desperate, place your mattress on the floor. If these methods level the mattress, but it is still too hard for comfort, try buying an extremely soft piece of one-inch foam rubber the size of your mattress, and see if the soft surface on your mattress allows you to sleep more comfortably.

IMPORTANT   You may find that a hard mattress actually does keep you more comfortable than a soft one. Use what makes your pain less!

Remember, the most important consideration is that you lessen your pain by allowing your back to learn to be free of pain. Use every possible method to achieve this end.

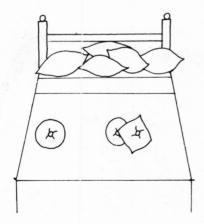

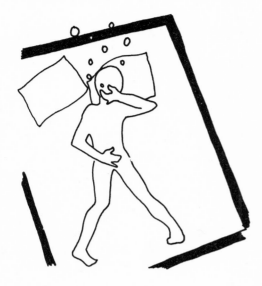

Waterbeds

A waterbed is very good for *most* people with low back problems. *Not for all!* There are always individuals who find that waterbeds actually give them a slight case of motion sickness or dizziness. *Don't ever use a waterbed if you are prone to motion sickness!* Your personal comfort is the most important thing to be considered. A case of motion sickness on top of low back pain can be the last straw. If you do not suffer from motion sickness, you may like to try a waterbed. Do not consider a waterbed if you have a low back problem and are sharing the bed with someone else. The changing tides as the other person shifts position will catch you un-prepared, and may cause you to tense up and experience more pain.

A heated waterbed can maintain your body at a higher temperature as you sleep. This prevents some stiffening of the back. The slight rhythmic movement of the waterbed, as it responds to your breathing, will also help keep the back supple.

The temperature of a waterbed can be adjusted. Your com-fort level becomes adjustable at your own hands, to some extent. A waterbed and Position #1, used together, should make a definite difference for you in a short period of time.

Use what is comfortable for you!

IMPORTANT   Do not use your waterbed as a large hot water bottle! Too much heat can leave you feeling very weak!

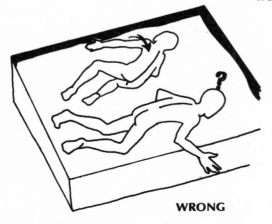

WRONG

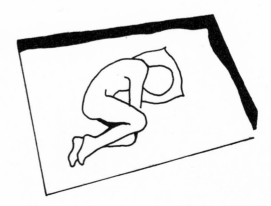

Making Beds

Use contoured sheets on your bed. Put one foot up on the bedframe when you change the linens. This will tilt your pelvis and help protect your back.

When you wake up in the morning, *stay in bed* and pull your top sheet up neatly. Slip out of bed without disturbing the sheets. *Don't* tuck in the sides! Use a wide comforter to cover the untucked sides.

If you feel that you must make beds and can't afford contoured sheets, throw a pillow on the floor. Use your hands on the edge of the bed for support, and lower yourself *slowly* onto one knee on the pillow.

Better yet — don't make the beds!

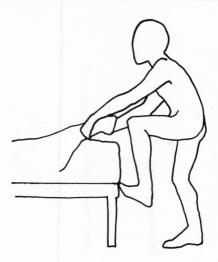

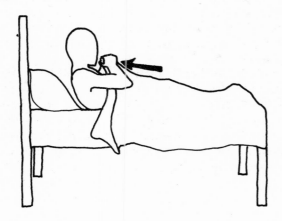

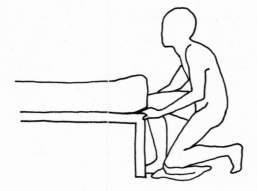

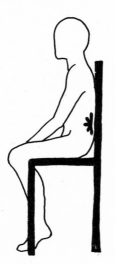

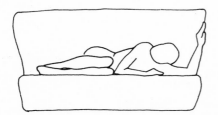

SITTING

IMPORTANT   Keep out of chairs and cars if you can, except for emergencies, like getting to the doctor!

You're either afraid of what will happen when you get up, or you have to *like* pain to sit if you don't absolutely have to when you have a back problem! For most people with low back pain, the only position more painful than sitting in a straight chair is (usually) sitting in a car.

In a car, you have the usual compression you get with sitting, plus the settling of parts for further compression (like coffee in a coffee can being shaken down) and on top of that double trouble, you have the pain of going over bumps, into potholes, around curves! If, in addition, you ride in a sports car, which has seats that are very low to the floor, you're in yet more trouble. If you must ride, lie down in the back seat. If you must drive, pull the seat forward so that your knees are bent. Place a rolled-up towel behind your bottom.

The chair that will give you the least trouble — the kind of chair that you should sit in if you must sit — is a rocking chair. Add a footstool, and a pillow behind your bottom, for further comfort. A rocking chair gives you the gentle rocking motion that will maintain circulation and keep your spine gently mobile. This, when you do get up, will allow you to move more easily.

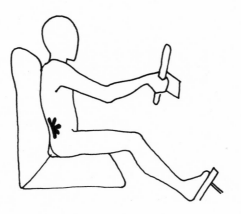

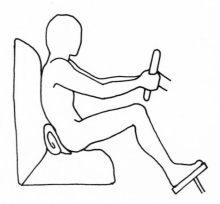

Sitting At a Desk

IMPORTANT   If you must sit in a straight chair at a desk to do your work, put all other objects you need on the other side of the room. Do not be efficient!

The longer you sit, the more you subject the discs of your lower back to compression. Get up often, take a minute to do the sink stretch, using your desk as the sink, and ease your back before you get your materials to continue your work. If you get up often enough to prevent the pain from occurring, you will be way ahead in your recovery.

Although getting out of the chair is best, there *are* ways to prevent pain or lessen it while you are sitting. Try putting a couple of thick phone books under your desk to rest your feet on. Those of you who have extreme lordosis must try other ways to relieve your tight backs before you can attempt the following position and do it properly.

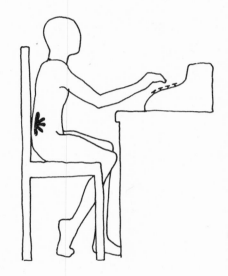

Modified Position #1 for Sitting

Many of the people you'll meet — in offices, in their homes — choose instinctively that position that makes their back most comfortable. Essentially it is Position #1 done in a sitting position.

IMPORTANT   All of the following maneuvers spread the body weight and reduce by 39.4 percent the large burden usually put on the lower back when you are sitting up straight.

Slump down onto your sacrum (that area of your back above your bottom that is bone covered with flesh), lean your shoulders back against the chair, and pick your legs up to rest them on the desk, the seat in front of you, across the arms of the chair, a table, anything that is handy. Have a pillow behind your bottom to support your lower back. No matter how comfortable positions may be, they all require fidgeting on your part. Shift often, even if it's only slightly. Your arms resting on the arms of a chair are a positive help in taking some pressure off the discs of your lower back.

It is better for your lower back if you get involved in work and pleasures that are more active than television-watching, movie-watching, and desk work. When you can — when

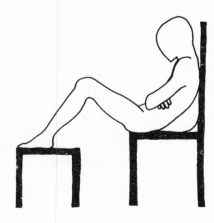

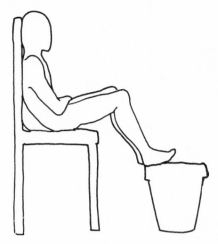

your back is free of pain and you can sit down on, and get back up from, the floor — it would be wise to rid your home of chairs, or to keep around only a few (as you keep some ashtrays) for those who cannot change, or do not wish to change, their habits!

This is *Modified Position* #1! No position in a chair will feel better for long, but this is the best you can do in a chair.

The position is great for sitting in movie theaters, also; put your feet or knees up on the back of the seat in front of you.

IMPORTANT   Whatever you do, don't think that because your back hurts you should sit down! Lie down if your back is hurting — in Position #1, if you can. Otherwise, keep out of the chair and do whatever exercises ease your back!

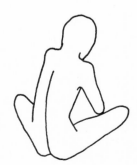

Sitting Without Crossing Your Legs

Crossing your legs creates a one-sided pull on your spine. If the crossed-leg position, favoring one side, gets to be a habit, the uneven compression can cause a more or less permanent distortion in your lower back.

Get up and move when you feel uncomfortable!

Most people cross their legs to ease the cutting-off of circulation in the back of the thigh that occurs when they sit in a chair with a poor seat. A better solution would be to put one or both legs up on a stool or a chair rung (not many of them around anymore!) or to get into the modified sitting position.

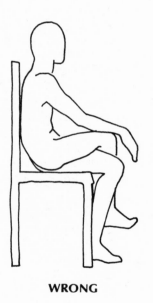

WRONG

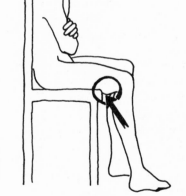

WRONG

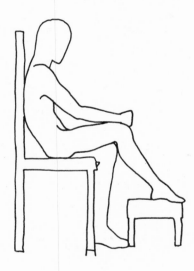

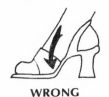

WRONG

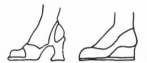

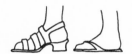

STANDING — FEET AND SHOES

We should all have great respect and admiration for our feet. With the proper treatment, our feet not only feel better, but they do their best for the rest of our body . . . and their best is quite something when you really look closely at them!

High heels: When your foot rests on a shoe with a heel, the front of your foot cannot work as it should. A high heel puts too much weight on the front of your foot, *narrows the base* (you use less of your foot), puts too much pressure on the crosswise arch, and makes ineffective the gripping action of your toes. If you are used to wearing high heels, be sure to change shoes so that you lower the height of the heels gradually over a period of weeks; this will prevent straining of the ligaments in your back and legs.

Wooden-soled shoes: We were given soft soles for a good reason. They prevent too great an impact on landing, especially on hard pavements and concrete floors. If anything, we need additional padding to protect us on impact. Rather than wearing shoes with wooden soles, try shoes with very soft crepe soles when you must walk in office buildings and on the streets.

Stiff shoes with a flat, hard sole: It is difficult for your entire foot to move from side to side at the ankle unless you pick it up off the floor, and even more difficult for the twenty-six bones in your feet to do their delicate job of balancing. The side-to-side balance is lost; the front-to-back balance is lost. The ability of your foot to contour itself to different surfaces is lost; the grasping ability of your toes is lost; the sensitivity of the sole, which enables it to determine different surfaces and textures, is lost.

What is most important is that, since you can't bend your

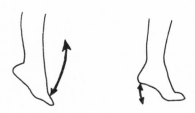
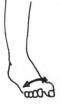
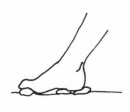
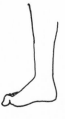

ankle because of the flat sole, the side-to-side balance is transported upward. This side-to-side balance, when transferred to your knee, can stretch knee ligaments, causing knee problems, especially if you are overweight! Women have a greater problem than men because of the angle of their thigh bone. Your knee is properly a hinge joint, providing back-and-forth movement with some rotation, which increases as the knee is bent. The side-to-side movement may be transferred up to your hips and even farther, to your lower back. Because of the distance from your feet, the compensating movements at the hips have to be much larger, side to side, than your lower back was built to take, especially if you are holding your hips stiff, to prevent pain. This may very well be part of your low back problem!

Minus heels: Lowering your heels with special shoes does a pretty good job of tilting your pelvis slightly and stretching your heel cords. For some problems, such as fallen metatarsals, they are useful. But a weak lower back that is simply tilted into position rather than strengthened into the tucked-pelvis position serves no long-term purpose! Your foot should be *flat* on the floor, with the flexibility and then the strength of the lower back adjusted until your body is taking care of itself as it was built to do, and as it will do if you treat it properly.

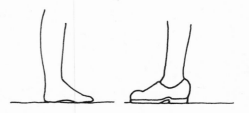

Try going barefoot as much as you can, and feel the difference in your back and in your balance. Walking this way will feel strange when you start. An embarrassment of riches! All those new movements and new sensations! It's a pity, but just as with too much of anything, you'll get over the newness of it and enjoy only the new ease with which you can move (at least around the house). Better soft-soled shoes for outside wear should be developed!

IMPORTANT   To help stop and to prevent low back pain, learn to wear only flexible, wide-front, soft, flat shoes with thick crepe soles
- **for less shortening of your back muscles;**
- **for less impact;**
- **for wider base;**
- **for better balance;**
- **for better grasp of toes!**

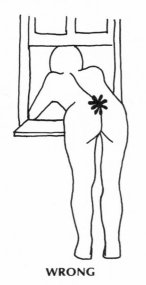

WRONG

BRUSHING TEETH AND OTHER WAIST-BENDERS

For brushing teeth, doing dishes, tending children, putting on a bra, washing your hair in a sink — do the *standing half-squat*.

Sometimes you will find yourself trapped into adopting the half-bend from the waist, which causes so much pain among those of you suffering with low back problems.

Think ahead! Anywhere that you know you are going to need this position to accomplish those necessary tasks, place a box or, better yet, a chair.

IMPORTANT   Putting one foot up on a box or a chair while standing will usually gain you a slight tipping forward of the pelvis. This will serve to hold your back in a better position, and spare you a lot of discomfort. Tighten your belly before lifting your leg!

Try different heights until you find the one that is most comfortable for you. Use whichever leg eases your back more. Try *both* the box and the chair — even putting one foot up on the side of the sink (if you have long legs and have become quite flexible). This also allows you to lean on your knee, lessening the strain still further.

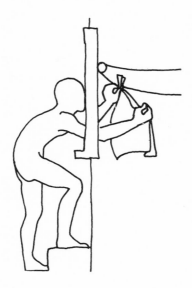

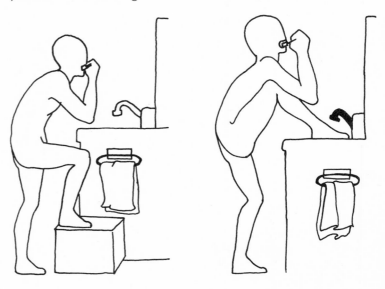

LIFTING

IMPORTANT   Lifting safely takes tight belly muscles! To get up from a squatting position safely, to get out of a chair, to lift a baby out of a crib, to pick up a heavy object from the floor or anywhere else, it is important to tighten the hip and back muscles, which control the flexing of the lumbar region (the tucking-under of the pelvis), and to stabilize that area by breathing out hard. As you do, remember to tighten your belly muscles!

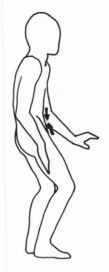

The whole effect is to have the back and belly held like a strung bow, the string being your belly muscles in front. This is really quite impossible for those of you with sway-back, or extreme lordosis. In practically every case, the extreme lordosis can be overcome by building those flexors of the back (the belly muscles, bottom muscles, and those that pull up the leg) to be strong enough to control the extensors (the long back muscles).

Your spine has over a hundred good strong muscular attachments to keep it strong. It takes positive attention to keep the many fewer opposing muscles — those toward the front — strong enough to equalize the strength from front to back. We are not living right — we no longer engage in the common daily activities that keep those muscles strong — or four out of five of us would not suffer low back pain at some time in our lives.

Learn to squat to pick up things from the floor without harming yourself. One foot placed behind the other *with your knees apart* makes squatting and lifting easier. You can test the weight and consistency of the object to be lifted by rocking it slightly from side to side. Finding you have hold of a bag of water whose contents roll from side to side, a box with a loose heavy object inside, which shifts suddenly, something much heavier than it looks — say, a small twenty-pound box of lead — will be a shock that your back should not have to react to suddenly. Testing the object with your hands first gives you the ability to judge more carefully how to handle it.

The next step is to pull the object in between your knees as close as possible to your body. Next, breathe out and tighten your belly muscles, tuck your bottom under and then pick up the object, keeping it as close to your body as

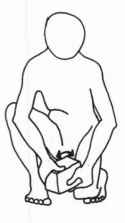

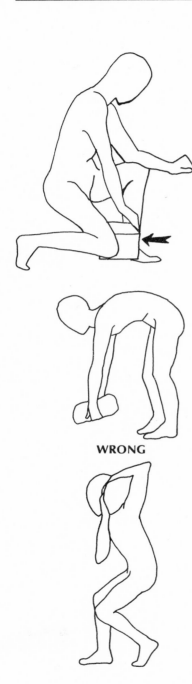

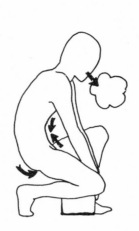

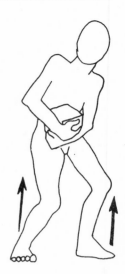

WRONG

you can. Now, breathing normally while holding your belly very tight you must rise straight up, using your thigh muscles, rather than leaning forward and putting the strain on your back!

IMPORTANT   If your thigh muscles are extremely weak (as many people's are), use the exercises from Chapter Six to build them back to usefulness! There is no other safe way to lift objects from the floor!

It may be best to shift the weight to your shoulder even *before* rising, so that you do not hold the weight in a position that may bother you.

To help prevent lasting deformities to the discs, it is wise to pick up the object, put it down at a more convenient level, then retighten your belly muscles and pick it up again for carrying.

This squatting method for lifting gives you more lifting power than does leaning over (which produces shearing stress) and reduces by far the number of low back injuries!

CARRYING

Carrying heavy burdens when your back is painful is a serious mistake. If you experience periodic pain in your back, it is best to leave carrying to others, or, at least, to wait until you have strengthened the basic structure of your back and learned how best to carry in order to relieve compression of the discs.

A basic rule for you if you have a "tricky" back should be — at the first sign of a twinge — either to put the load down or to readjust it! Try never to carry a package in front of you. Just placing it there makes you readjust backward from your waist. This will encourage compression and pain.

IMPORTANT   A heavy load carried on one side can cause leaning to one side. This will encourage compression and pain. If you must carry to one side, lift your other arm out to the side to counterbalance the load. Do not lean to the side when carrying!

Carrying an equal amount of weight on each side relieves the problem somewhat, but the best solution, if you must carry, is to place the object on your shoulders. A yoke for carrying would be ideal, but lacking that, just place the burden slightly forward on your shoulder and hold it in place with your hand. Your muscles will tend to push *up* toward it,

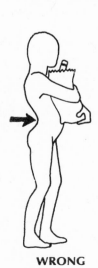

WRONG

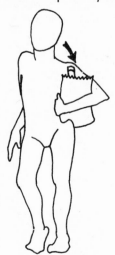

WRONG

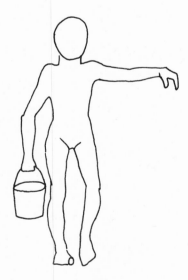

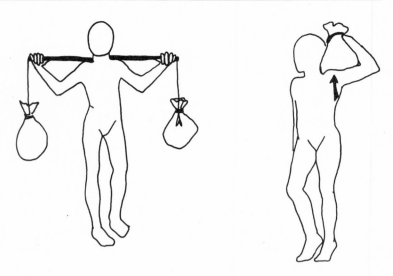

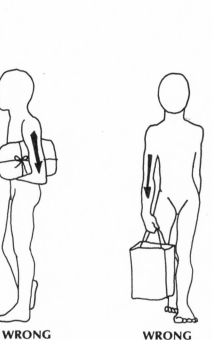

WRONG   **WRONG**

rather than — as when you have it hanging from your hands or tucked under your arms —to pull down.

IMPORTANT   **Soft, thick-soled, flat shoes that are not high around the ankle will really pay off for you if you must carry loads often. Keeping your knees bent and easy in movement will help to take some of the shock of extra compression and impact off your lower back. If the package is to be carried any distance, stopping often to stretch will help. (Put the load down first!) Always keep your belly muscles tight while lifting and carrying!**

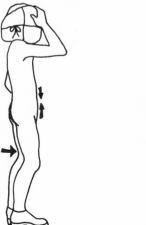

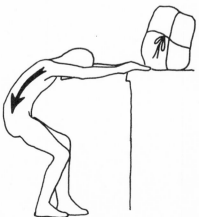

TAKING DOWN FROM AND PUTTING UP OVERHEAD

While your back is still in pain, let someone else do the putting up and taking down! When your back is better, arrange to do it safely.

Take off your shoes (for better balance at a lower level — foot level — to lessen any chances of falling). Stand on two chairs placed front to front. (These chairs should be placed on a rubber mat so that they cannot slip.) The chair backs give you something to hold on to while you get up and down; this is especially important if you tend to lose your balance. The two chairs also provide you with a wider base of support than a single chair.

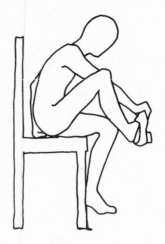

One foot should be on one chair and the other foot on the other chair. Keep your feet turned out and far enough apart so that you feel comfortably balanced. Be sure your back is in the proper position, your pelvis curled under, knees bent, belly really tight. Hold that position throughout any lifting or lowering and placing. Whatever you are either putting up or taking down from a high shelf is going to have a horizontal force. It will slide either toward you or away from you, according to the direction of the force you apply. One foot must be back, one forward, to give you leeway in movement without any loss of balance.

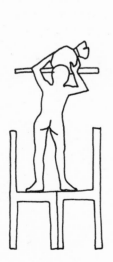
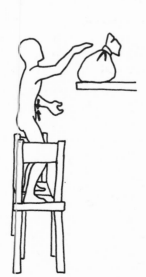
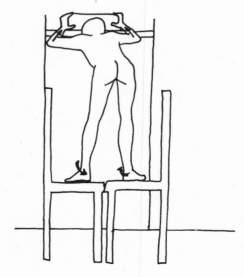

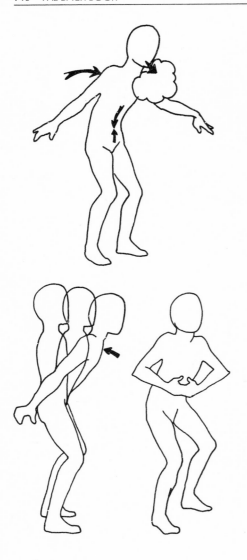

If your right foot is forward, your left hand should be used for pushing or pulling and your right hand for stabilizing. Check to see which foot forward makes you feel most secure in your balance.

If heights bother you at all, it helps to push a table over close to the chairs. This gives you a greater feeling of security. Look toward the table rather than toward the floor if you must look down during the operation of lifting or lowering.

SNEEZING, COUGHING, LAUGHING, VOMITING

When your body is thrown uncontrollably forward, hold this extreme position, especially immediately at the end of the convulsive movement.

Tighten your belly muscles as you are thrown foward, and hold them *tight* (to prevent the "fly-back" effect)!

This should prevent most of the discomfort.

Let the relaxation of the muscles, as you move from the extreme position, happen slowly and gradually, always under your control.

Laced Fingers

If you have very weak belly muscles, lacing your fingers across your belly and holding them there tightly can ease your back when you are rising or defecating or coughing or laughing or sneezing or throwing up.

This laced-finger pressure is handmade belly muscle support, to be used until you make your own belly muscles strong enough to do their job!

SAFE POSITIONS FOR SEXUAL INTERCOURSE

It is better not to force the information on positions for sexual intercourse on your spouse or sex partner!

If your partner hasn't found a way, you may have missed a message!

We each have different pain levels that we find bearable. Some of us seem to be able to stand pain in one part of the body better than in another part. Some of us *think* we can — none of us really can — judge how much pain another person is having or how much he or she can stand. Some people go into shock with a small amount of pain; others can climb out of a car wreck with broken bones, and walk away.

If someone tells you that his or her back is hurting too much to be able either to perform or enjoy sexual intercourse, *believe it!* One bad performance can trigger a whole series of poor performances, and may eventually, by creating fear or embarrassment, form a habit you will not want to live with. The psychological aspects of intercourse are well known, but are poorly understood or dealt with. Leave well enough alone.

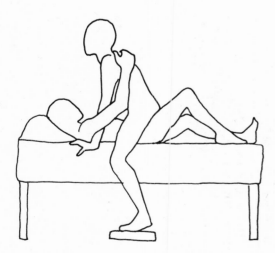 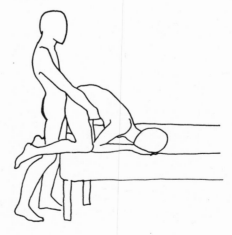

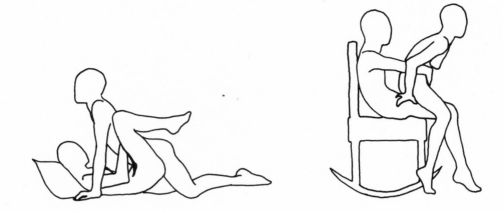

In the meantime, those of you with partners who let nothing stand in their way can try these safe positions, illustrated in the pictures.

IMPORTANT   The person who is not in pain should be the one to provide the action in sexual intercourse.

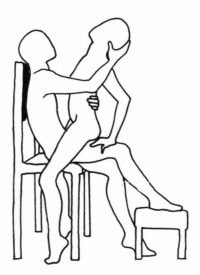

FLYING

You should not fly during an acute attack of pain!

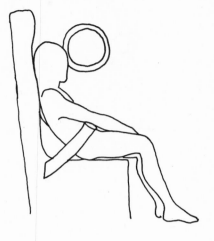

The shearing forces on your lower vertebrae go up as the plane accelerates along the ground. Then, as the plane lifts, the forces of compression add to the shear until the plane gains its final speed and reaches the altitude at which it will cruise.

In case you do take an airplane trip, try to get a seat in the first forward row of whichever class you ride, or else in a row that gives some leg room. Then you can slump enough with your seat belt buckled so that your pelvis is pointed somewhat to the front of the plane. This will relieve, though probably not completely, the pain you may feel during takeoff.

Don't ride elevators either, if you can help it. Try escalators or stairs. If you must use elevators, take the basic standing position, Modified Position #1, with your bottom tucked under and your knees bent, and tighten your belly as much as you can — or back up to the wall of the elevator in this position and lean your waistline against the wall with your feet out a little way. Either of these two ways of standing will give you some relief.

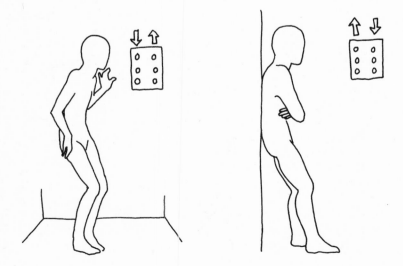

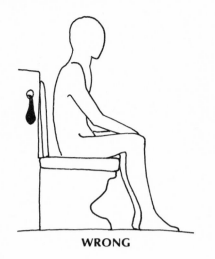

WRONG

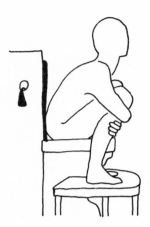

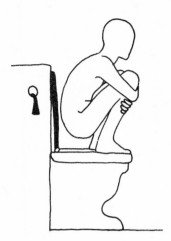

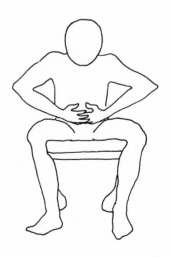

TOILETS

You must find a different way of sitting on the toilet, especially if your back is hurting. The way you sit now leaves your belly muscles unsupported, as they would be by your thighs if you were squatting. It leaves your lower back uncurled, as it would be if you were squatting in a protecting position. You should put a stool in front of the toilet upon which you can rest your feet, or, better yet, a u-shaped stool around the toilet so that your feet can be your total support and your back is really curved and protected, or you can — don't laugh, this is a serious suggestion — squat on the toilet seat itself!

It has been proven that people defecating in a squatting position even manage to pass a larger stool — not surprising, when you think about how much better a position this is. It would allow you to empty yourself more completely and would decrease your back's tendency to ache.

Many of us cannot squat because we lack practice. You should be able to. You still can learn to squat. At least you can support your belly wall by grabbing hold of one wrist with the other hand, or lacing your fingers, and exerting counterpressure with your hands against the lower belly wall while you are having a bowel movement.

SPORTS AND DANCES TO AVOID

It is difficult for me to give you this advice.

IMPORTANT All body-contact and impact sports should be avoided if you have a low back problem. Any dancing that includes jumps should also be avoided.

Now that you've been given the advice, let me make a suggestion for those of you who choose to ignore it — which you shouldn't. Before and after indulging in your favorite activity (also during, if you cause yourself pain), get into Position #1 or one of the other *stretch* positions. The stretch positions will help to undo the further damage you are doing to your lower back with compression, impact, and twisting.

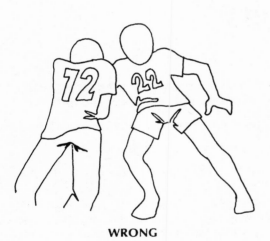

WRONG

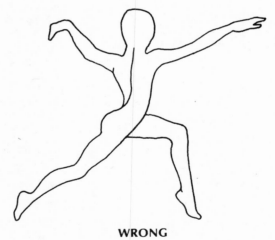

WRONG

ELEVEN

Exercises to Avoid

If you are going to do other exercises before you are ready, at least protect yourself by these few rules of thumb!

First: Do not cause yourself more pain than you have!

Second: Do no exercises that arch your back!

The exercise shown here compresses the edge of the disc and is responsible for causing much unnecessary pain. Lifting either one or both ends of your body is wrong. Both ends at once can be twice as bad! There are alternate ways to strengthen your back muscles. See Chapter Four, Position #2.

Third: Do no exercises that cause you to lift your legs against gravity.

Lifting up your legs against gravity when your belly muscles are weak makes your back tend to come up into an arch. Even if this does not cause pain (which would be surprising!), it does prolong the very problems you should be trying to overcome. There are safer and better ways to de-

146

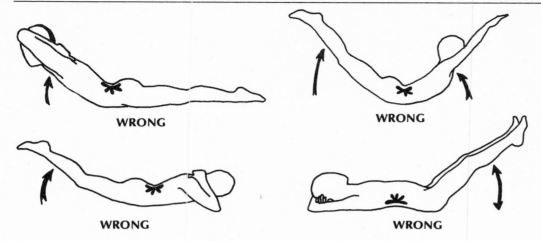

WRONG
WRONG
WRONG
WRONG

velop lower belly strength with your pelvis stabilized in the right position. See Chapter Four, Position #2.

Fourth: When it is possible to avoid them, do no exercises that allow compression.

Don't do any exercises standing up if you can do them while you're lying down, thereby relieving the stress of gravity on your spine.

Note: You may be one-half to one inch taller lying down than you are when standing. All that extra extension is in the disc material. Lying down lessens compression and the chance of pain. Your knees should be bent to begin. See Chapter Four, Position #2.

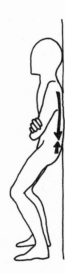

Fifth: There are a number of reasons why a traditional exercise for low back problems can be quite bad. Let's go into them.

1. When the knee-to-chest move is first initiated, lifting your knees toward your chest rather than picking them up with your hands puts your lower back under strain.

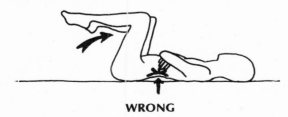

WRONG

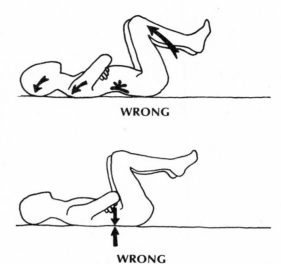

WRONG

WRONG

2. If your head is on the floor, especially when you begin to lift your knees, the tendency is to use the back of your head and your shoulders to press into the floor. This tightens the muscles down your back, fighting the flexibility — the curve — that you are trying to develop.

3. The position of your back prevents you from developing the flexibility in just that part of your lower back where you need it, because that part is held in place by the surface of the bed.

4. If you have your hands around rather than behind your knees, you may overstretch the tissues of your knee, which need to be stretched gently and slowly. This will give you additional problems.

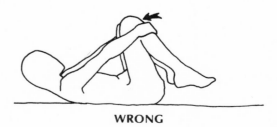

WRONG

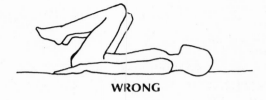

WRONG

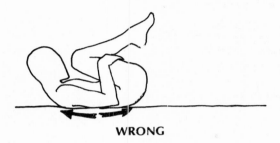

WRONG

5. Many people have hip joints that can become very flexible without the pelvis ever moving. This means that the low back area, in this position, may never get one bit more flexible.

6. Pulling your knees in tight stretches too far that tissue that is under a strain. The extreme stretching can cause tearing within the tissue or can even pull the tissue loose from its attachments on the bone.

7. Bouncing your knees toward your chest, rather than easing them and relaxing them from the chest, can really be painful if you have irritated or swollen tissue. (If you had a bad burn on one arm, close to your wrist, that you could see and feel, and you wanted to put on an expanding watch band, would you let it snap into place or would you ease it to your wrist very gently?) Any movement where there is swollen or irritated tissue must be made cautiously, repeated as seldom as possible while still giving results, so as not to cause more pain!

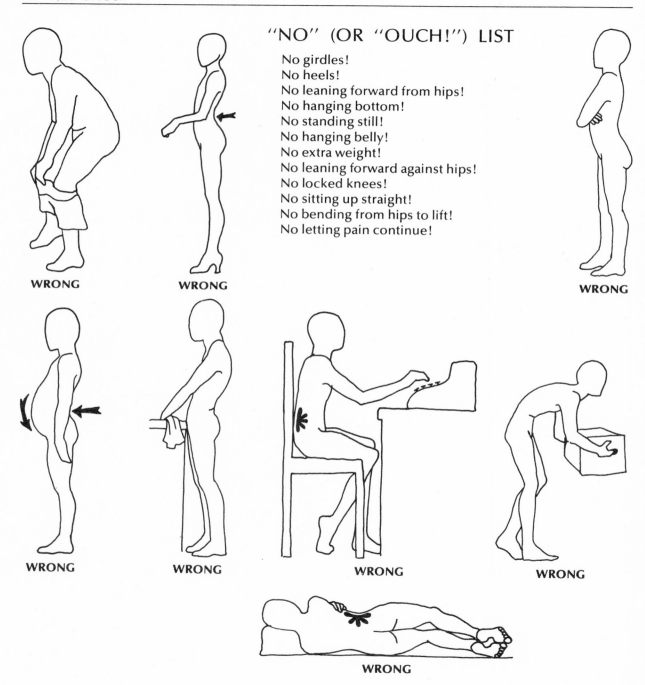

"NO" (OR "OUCH!") LIST

No girdles!
No heels!
No leaning forward from hips!
No hanging bottom!
No standing still!
No hanging belly!
No extra weight!
No leaning forward against hips!
No locked knees!
No sitting up straight!
No bending from hips to lift!
No letting pain continue!

WRONG

WRONG

WRONG

WRONG

WRONG

WRONG

WRONG

WRONG

TWELVE

Your Maintenance Program

YOUR MAINTENANCE PROGRAM

There is very little that you need to continue to do to keep your lower back healthy. Once you have freed yourself of pain and rebuilt your strength in such a way as to hold your pelvis in the proper position, you need only two or three exercises to act as reminders and to keep the muscles strong.

IMPORTANT   From this day forward, habit becomes your most important asset!

If you use the proper standing position, if you make your belly rigid before any lifting, carrying, or getting up, if you maintain strong belly and thigh muscles — there may be no reason for you to experience low back pain again.

Use the other reminders for insurance!

TILT! TIGHTEN! CLENCH!

IMPORTANT   Tilt your pelvis. Tighten your belly. Clench your bottom. When you tilt your pelvis, purse your mouth

151

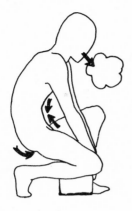

and breathe out hard to tighten your belly. Keep it tight and then breathe normally. And clench your bottom!

If you can remember to tilt your pelvis, tighten your belly hard, and clench your bottom *before* beginning any lifting; during any carrying; any time you are lying on your back and need to stretch out or pull in or pull up your legs, you can prevent an enormous number of painful incidents with your lower back!

Tightening your belly almost always results in pulling your pelvis under and reduces the forces on the fifth lumbar disc by 30 percent! A rigid belly stabilizes the belly muscles so that your back can move safely — and often without any pain!

Tilt! Tighten! Clench! Practice doing these three before each move!

WHEN YOUR BACK IS IN PAIN

IMPORTANT   After a low back flare-up or whenever your back is in pain, use only Position #1 until most of the pain is gone!

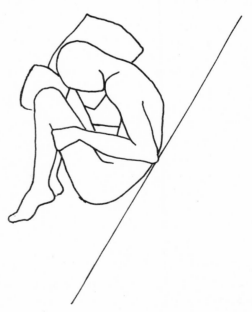

POSITION #1

Once you can ease your knees to your nose, or once you get as close as you can and feel reasonably comfortable sleeping in that position nightly — once you are free of pain — there is no reason to become puritanical about retaining the strict form of Position #1 throughout the entire night.

Try once before you go to sleep to get your knees and nose close together — and in the morning just before arising, again try to get your knees and your nose close together — just to be sure that you can do it.

IMPORTANT   Do Position #1 slowly every time! Add on the breathing and relaxing every time! Undo it slowly every time!

The rest of the night, try to retain some semblance of that position, keeping your waistline *rounded out!* Keep your chin tucked in toward your chest, of course, and your knees at least slightly forward.

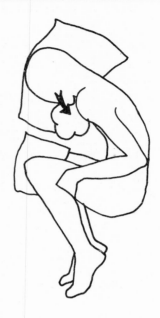

POSITION #2

All muscles used in Position #2 should be strong enough and practiced enough so that you can maintain this position, when standing, more comfortably than your old posture.

Take the time to acquire a good standing posture in Position #2.

Now continue to practice Position #2 in bed just once a day — paying close attention to every point — for as many minutes as you can. Tilt! Tighten! Clench! Keep your chin toward your chest! Keep your feet turned up toward your knees!

Do a few intermittent sink, rolling, or overhead bar stretches afterward. All stretches should be done as stretch-relax-stretch-relax-stretch-relax — one after the other.

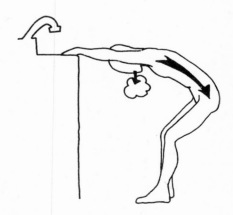

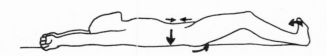

ROLLING STRETCHES

Extending the disc material every day is an excellent idea, if only to fight gravity and the compression of the discs caused by lifting and carrying.

Try stretching repeatedly, especially in the afternoons and evenings, when the day-long effect of gravity will have taken its toll — making you shorter, less comfortable, and stiffer in movement.

Try stretching, if it is convenient, each time you have lifted or carried something. Grab hold of a sink, stretch slowly backward, with your bottom and head tucked under, your knees bent. Repeat the stretch several times. When you feel relaxed, start moving from your hips *gently*, to get more movement in your hip joints and more stretch in your lower back.

Continuing this movement each time you stretch, slowly round your lower back. Continue the movement up your spine until you are standing. Then begin again.

Try repeating these rolling stretches several times — maybe 3 or 4 times a day. More is fine!

Use the rolling stretches, which combine sink stretches, hip flexibility, and rolling stretches. Or, if it feels better for you and is convenient, do the overhead bar stretches.

IMPORTANT   All stretches are improved by being repeated at least three times. More is better. Be gentle but be consistent.

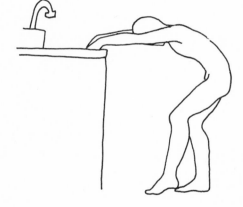

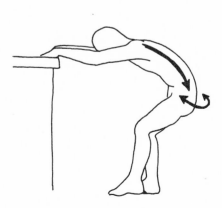

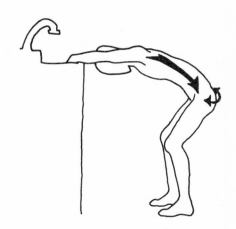

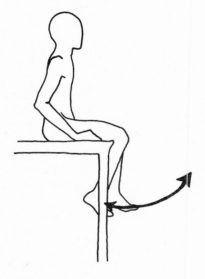
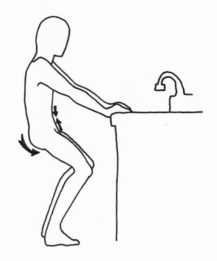
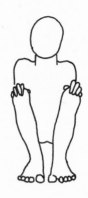

POSITION #3

This check list is to be used after you have worked your way up to — and have again gotten back to — squatting comfortably.

Sit on the edge of a table — or just stand and swing your lower leg 30 times from the knee.

Then, still standing —
Tilt! Tighten! Clench!
— and slowly squat!
— leaning very slightly forward;
— preferably barefoot;
— knees moving out over your feet.
Tilt! Tighten! Clench!
— and, leaning slightly forward,
slowly rise!
Do this *at least* 5 or 6 times each day!

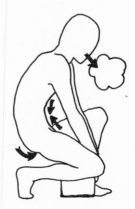

FIDGETING — SMALL EASING MOVES

Whether you are standing, sitting, or lying down, *you do yourself an injury when you stop moving!*

Your whole system is built to move, to grow, according to how you move; to circulate your blood, oxygen, and food, according to how you move; to develop strength in your muscles and bones, according to how you move. *An absence of movement will automatically allow your body to begin deteriorating.*

Your various internal systems lose their synchrony of movement when you stop moving. You stop depositing the building materials that come into your body in the form of food because your body does not have need of them in the same amounts when you stop moving. Your bones weaken and break easily; your muscles atrophy and hang (especially your belly and bottom!); your veins bulge; breathing becomes shallow; blood pressure does not readjust properly, making you dizzy on sudden movement. Your connective tissues stiffen, making you less easy in movement. Your balance slowly becomes worse and worse, as mechanisms for balance are left un- or little used.

Use rocking chairs or Modified Position #1 whenever you are sitting. Shift from foot to foot while standing, and if you are in bed — especially while in Position #1 — use small easing moves to redistribute yourself, always staying within the boundaries of comfort!

IMPORTANT   Do not cause yourself pain, but keep moving as much as possible!

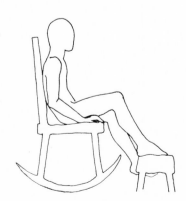

OVERALL REMINDER LIST

1. Prevent jamming.
2. Sleep in Position #1 —
   adjust carefully!
3. Position #2 — tighten belly and bottom to tuck and tilt
   pelvis. Tighten belly and tuck pelvis under to
   > walk;
   > squat;
   > get up;
   > carry;
   > lift;
   > stand — don't stand still!
   >> always stand with knees unlocked!
4. Use intermittent stretching from sink or bar.
5. Keep your back warm.
6. Lift and lower loads only with spine held vertically.
7. Put one foot on box when bending forward slightly.
8. Go barefoot or wear soft shoes with thick, soft crepe
   soles.
9. Sit in Modified Position #1.
   Use floor for sitting; "no hands" rising!

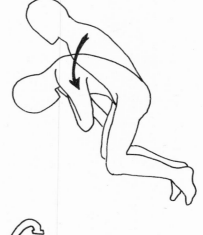

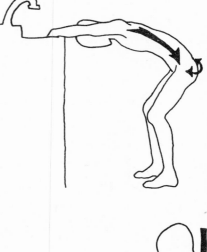

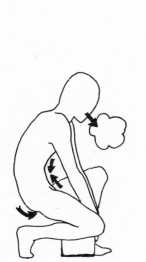

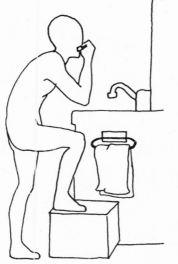

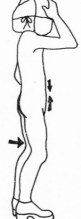

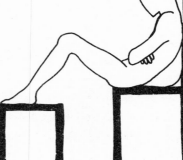

Bibliography

Basmajian, J. V. *Grant's Method of Anatomy* 8th ed. Baltimore: Williams and Wilkins Company, 1975.

Becker, Frederick R., James Wilson, John A. Gehweiler. *The Anatomical Basis of Medical Practice*. Baltimore: Williams and Wilkins Company, 1971.

Cailliet, Rene. *Low Back Pain Syndrome*. 2nd ed. Philadelphia: F. A. Davis Company, 1974.

Ciba Foundation Symposium 8 (New Series). *Physiology, Emotion and Psychosomatic Illness*. Elsevier Exerpta Medica, North-Holland. Amsterdam, London, and New York: Associated Scientific Publishers, 1972.

Damon, Albert, Howard W. Stoudt, and Ross A. McFarland. *The Human Body in Equipment Design*. 2nd ed. Cambridge, Mass: Harvard University Press, 1971.

Edholm, D. G. *The Biology of Work*. New York and Toronto: World University Library, McGraw-Hill Book Company, 1967.

Hytten, Frank E. and Isabella Leitch. *The Physiology of Human Pregnancy*. Oxford, England: Blackwell Scientific Publications, 1964.

Johnson, Perry B., Wynn F. Updyke, Donald C. Stolberg, and Maryellen Schaefer. *Physical Education: A Problem-Solving Approach to Health and Fitness*. New York: Holt, Rinehart and Winston, 1966.

Kendall, Henry O., Florence P. Kendall, and Gladys E. Wadsworth. *Muscles, Testing and Function*. 2nd ed. Baltimore: Williams and Wilkins Company, 1975.

Krusen, Frank H., ed., Kottke, Frederick J. and Paul M. Elwood, associate eds. *Handbook of Physical Medicine and Rehabilitation*. 2nd ed. Philadelphia, London, and Toronto: W. B. Saunders Company, 1971.

Licht, Sidney, ed. *Rehabilitation and Medicine*. Baltimore: Waverly Press, Inc., 1968.

Michele, Arthur A. *Iliopsoas — Development of Anomalies in Man*. Springfield, Illinois: Charles C. Thomas, 1962.

Rasch, Philip J., Roger K. Burke. *Kineseology and Applied Anatomy: The Science of Human Movement*. 3rd ed. Philadelphia: Lea and Febiger, 1968.

Ruch, Theodore C. and Harry D. Patton, eds. *Physiology and Biophysics*. 19th ed. Philadelphia and London: W. B. Saunders Company, 1966.

Schleyer-Saunders, E. *Backache in Women*. Bristol, England: John Wright and Sons Ltd., 1966.

Steindler, Arthur. *Kineseology of the Human Body, Under Normal and Pathological Conditions*. Springfield, Illinois: Charles C. Thomas, 1964.

Van Cott, Harold P. and Robert G. Kinkade, eds. Joint Army–Navy–Air Force Steering Committee, sponsors. *Human Engineering Guide to Equipment Design*. Revised ed. Washington, D.C.: American Institutes for Research, 1972.

Wells, Katherine F. *Kineseology: The Scientific Basis of Human Motion*. 4th ed. Philadelphia and London: W. B. Saunders Company, 1969.

Williams, Paul C. *Low Back and Neck Pain*. Springfield, Illinois: Charles C. Thomas, 1974.

Williams, Paul C. *The Lumbosacral Spine — Emphasizing Conservative Management*. New York, Toronto, Sydney, and London: Blakiston Division, McGraw-Hill Book Company, 1965.